homoeopathy of the
mercury

Dr Yubraj Sharma

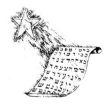

published by academy of light

The material in this book is freely available to copy for teaching and demonstration purposes provided the author is acknowledged in an appropriate manner, but cannot be used for re-sale, hire or otherwise circulated in any form (including electronic) without the publisher's prior consent.

First published in the UK in 2003 by Academy of Light Ltd

ISBN 1-904472-00-1

British Library Cataloguing in-Publication Data.
A catalogue record of this book is available from the British Library.

The right of Dr Yubraj Sharma to be identified as Author of this work has been asserted by him in accordance with the Copyright, Designs and Patents Act, 1998.

Text: © Dr Yubraj Sharma 2003
Illustrations: © Katherine Mynott 2003
Design: Bumblebee, 5 Nelson Road, Greenwich, London SE10 9JB

Printed in the United Kingdom by BFS Printing Ltd

Published by Academy of Light Ltd
Unit 1c Delta Centre, Mount Pleasant, Wembley,
Middlesex HA0 1UX, UK
Tel: 0044 (0)20 8795 2695 Fax: 0044 (0)20 8903 3748

This book is lovingly dedicated to fellow lightworkers
and all my brothers and sisters on Earth.

I offer a special dedication to Mita Shah for her support,
and Silvie Turner without whom this book would not
have come to manifest.

It is written in honour of Mercury for accompanying
the evolutionary journey of humanity and
in gratitude to all the spiritual beings
constantly assisting my medical work.

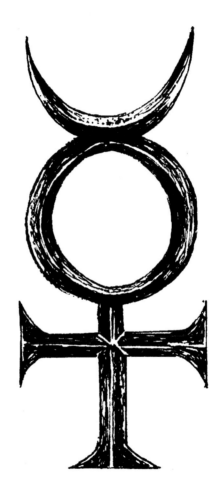

Astrological glyph of Mercury the planet.

contents

permissions	i
table of figures	ii
table of symbols	iv
introduction	v
chapter 1: basic overview	**1**
spiritual formation of the solar system planets	1
mercury vapour on earth	1
breathing process and astrality	2
lemuria and the development of consciousness	3
basic spiritual theme of the remedy	4
chapter 2: homoeopathic picture	**6**
mercurius solubilis	7
mentals	*7*
temperature	*9*
sexuality	*10*
breathing processes	*10*
inflammation	*10*
perspiration and discharges	*10*
anti-syphilitic	*11*
mercurius corrosivus	11
mentals	*12*
generals	*12*
particulars	*12*
mercurius iodatus flavus	*12*
mentals	*13*
generals	*13*
particulars	*13*
the elements of the periodic table	*13*
mercurius iodatus ruber	15

CONTENTS

mercurius oxycyanide	15
mentals	16
particulars	16
spiritual theme of the remedy	16
chapter 3: mercury as metal	18
metal and planet relationship	18
relationship with old saturn and lead	18
mining of mercury	19
cinnabar ore	20
properties of liquid mercury	22
properties of mercury light	24
mercury and the atmosphere	25
chemical catalytic properties	27
chapter 4: toxic effects of mercury poisoning	29
forms and uses of mercury	29
absorption of mercury	31
distribution of mercury after absorption	31
toxic effects	31
symptoms of toxic poisoning	32
chapter 5: cosmological principles	34
septenary division of all bodies	34
nebulae theory of the solar system	38
formation of mercury after old sun separation from earth	40
chapter 6: mercury's astronomical properties	42
orbit and rotation	42
orbit around the sun	42
conjunctions during orbit	45
rotational speed and relationship with the orbital speed	47
sun retrograde, double sunset and double sunrise	48
relationship with the moon orbit	52
temperature fluctuations due to orbit and rotation	52
evolution of the rotational speed	53
surface appearance	54

CONTENTS

iron core and magnetic field ... 57
the atmosphere ... 59

chapter 7: mercury and the cabalah of number ... 62
gematria ... 62
   logos ... 63
   god self ... 64
   a soul ... 66
   pillar ... 67
   gilgul ... 67

chapter 8: mercury in astrology and psychology ... 68
basic themes ... 68
mercury retrograde ... 69
personality types when mercury is direct in the natal chart ... 73
personality types when mercury is retrograde in the natal chart ... 73
planetary rulership of zodiacal signs ... 74
   gemini ... 76
   virgo ... 76
   aries ... 77
   scorpio ... 77

chapter 9: mercury in mythology ... 79
manifestations of mercury ... 79
   mythology of gemini ... 79
the works of homer ... 80
birth of mercury ... 80
the god of travel ... 82
the caduceus ... 83
   the coiled snakes ... 84
   the pranic tube ... 85
the messenger of the gods ... 86
   the scattering of souls ... 86
   humanity's need for guidance ... 88
   the fates ... 88
   the ibis form of thoth ... 90
the death process ... 92

CONTENTS

the daimon of fate	93
thoth and ancient egypt	94
guide to the dead souls, the psychopomp	96
hades the underworld	97
ruler of thieves and liars	98
ruler of discovering and finding	101
music and venus	103
mercury in myth and language	105
mercury and sexuality in myth	105
asclepius and the greco-roman temples of healing	107
kabeirean mysteries and the fallen angels	111
overall character of the god	113

chapter 10: mercury and the human personality — 115

mercury and forgetting	115
stability of the personality	121
thinking	121
viewing the outside world	121
ownership of thoughts	121
history of thinking	122
third-dimensional thinking	122
multidimensional thinking	124
transcendentalism (mercury)	124
the throat chakra	124

chapter 11: mercury within the human civilisation — 128

mercury in the atlantean age	128
mercury in ancient egypt	130
ancient gold and silver refining	132
alchemical uses of mercury	135
ancient and modern therapeutic uses of mercury	139
pink disease	139
autism	140
amalgam fillings in dentistry	141
syphilis, aids and hiv	142
overcoming toxicity in the chakras	142
mercury and mad hatter disease	143

CONTENTS

production of mirrors with mercury and tin ... 143
contemporary medical and scientific uses of mercury ... 144

chapter 12: mercury in the biological and cellular realm ... 148
the relationship between cells and the whole organism ... 148
diseases due to cellular separation ... 149
influence on digestion ... 151
mercury and syphilis ... 153
    the nature of bacteria and the spirochetes ... 153
    homoeopathic miasms ... 154
    general morphology and motility of spirochete bacteria ... 155
    morphology of treponema pallidum ... 157
    pathogenesis and immunity of syphilis ... 162
    epidemiology of syphilis ... 166

chapter 13: mercury in breathing and circulation ... 169
inspiration/inhalation ... 169
exhalation ... 169
astral body incarnation and the state of soul ... 171
mercury and iron forces ... 175
the spiritual significance of human blood ... 175
heart and lung circulation ... 179

chapter 14: occult anatomy and the hermaphrodite nature ... 182
the brain and reproductive organs ... 184
the root races and procreation ... 186
syphilis and the lemurian age ... 189
sexual energy distortions ... 192
sexual evolution and the influence of the seventh ray ... 197
the chakras and sexual energy ... 202

chapter 15: mercury and old saturn in the skeletal anatomy ... 206
the clavicles ... 206
uprightness and the el-shift ... 208
the snake and the human pranic tube ... 209
the cosmic lemniscate form ... 211
the skeleton and saturn forces ... 212

CONTENTS

chapter 16: mercury and dental anthropology   215

structure of a tooth   217
the concept of species in spiritual dental anthropology   218
the giants   222
odontoglyphics   224
malocclusion of teeth   225
    diastema   226
    irregular rotation and winging of teeth   227
    impacted teeth   230
    congenitally absent teeth   231
    supernumerary teeth   232
    retention of milk teeth   232
sequence and timing of dental growth   233
dental enamel   234
    hypoplasia of enamel   236
    opacities and hypocalcifications   236
    dental fluorosis and staining of teeth   236
    syphilitic teeth changes   239
    anthropological studies   239

final thoughts   240

glossary   241

bibliography   263

index   264

permissions

I have listed the permissions granted by other publishing bodies for extracts and use of materials from their works, received with thanks.

Edelstein, Emma Jeanette and Ludwig. 'Asclepias: A Collection and Interpretation of the Testimonies', Vol I & II. Extract from 'Inscriptiones Graecae' IV, 1, 121-2, Stele I 'Cures of Apollo and Asclepius' (ET 423) and extract by Elder Pliny, 'Natural History', XXV, 4(11), (30) (ET 369) © 1945. [Copyright Holder]. Reprinted with permission of the John Hopkins University Press.

Hart, Gerald D. 'Asclepias: the God of Medicine' pp.82, 83. © 2000. The Royal Society of Medicine Press Ltd. Reprinted with permission the above extracts subject to primary permission of the John Hopkins University Press [Copyright Holder].

Kerenyi, Karl. 'Hermes: Guide of Souls' pp.41, 53, 55, 56, 58, 61, 63, 67, 77, 78, 83 translated extracts from Homer's 'Odyssey', 'Illiad' and 'Hymn'. © 1976. [Copyright Holder]. Reprinted with permission of Spring Publications Inc.

Hillson, Simon. 'Dental Anthropology' pp.7, 11, 108. Artistic reproductions of illustrations for figures 16.1, 16.2, 16.3 and 16.4 in this work. © 1996. [Copyright Holder]. Reproduced with permission of Cambridge University Press.

table of figures

Cover illustration the god Mercury

Fig. 2-1.	Table of Mercury chemical compounds	6
Fig. 5-1.	The ten planetary schemes of evolution within the solar system	35
Fig. 5-2.	Earth chain with seven rounds	36
Fig. 6-1.	Oscillation of Mercury to the left and right of the Sun when seen from the Earth's perspective	43
Fig. 6-2.	Visibility of Mercury above the (a) eastern and (b) western horizon	43
Fig. 6-3.	Visible path of Mercury when combined with the movement of the Sun along the horizon	44
Fig. 6-4.	Appearances of Mercury in the east during the morning (before sunrise), and the west during the evening (after sunset) over the course of the year	44
Fig. 6-5.	Spiralling curves of Mercury's combined path as a caduceus	44
Fig. 6-6.	Mercury's synodical orbit around the Sun with conjunctions during one Earth year	46
Fig. 6-7.	Mercury's rotation/orbit ratio of 3:2 around the Sun	47
Fig. 6-8.	Movement of the Sun as seen on Mercury at perihelion and sub-solar maximal point	49
Fig. 6-9.	Double sunset at 90° east of solar maximal point at perihelion around the Sun	50
Fig. 6-10.	Double sunrise at 90° west of solar maximal point at perihelion around the Sun	51
Fig. 6-11.	Comparison of the Moon's synodical orbit with the orbit of Mercury	53
Fig. 7-1.	Table of gematria alpha numbers for the English alphabet	62
Fig. 7-2.	Nature of self as monad, personality and intervening soul	65
Fig. 7-3.	Spiralling energies of varying stages of integration between monad and personality	66
Fig. 8-1.	Table of planetary levels of rulership for Mercury in astrology	75
Fig. 9-1.	Caduceus of Mercury with two spiralling serpents	83
Fig. 9-2.	Ibis form of Thoth	91
Fig. 9-3.	Anubis, an incarnation of Thoth	95
Fig. 10-1.	Larynx (voicebox) anterior view	125

TABLE OF FIGURES

Fig. 12-1.	Syphilis bacterium, Treponema pallidum: (a) microscopic, (b) expanded microscopic view, (c) transverse section showing position of endoflagella	156
Fig. 12-2.	Spiritual energies involved in movement of Treponema pallidum at two walls and endoflagella	158
Fig. 12-3.	(a) Symbol for the 'I Ching', (b) comparison of 'I Ching' with chromosomal double-stranded DNA	160
Fig. 13-1.	Respiratory system with depiction of astral flow	170
Fig. 13-2.	Portion of a lung lobule showing alveoli and Mercury process	171
Fig. 14-1.	Cerebrum and brainstem	183
Fig. 15-1.	Clavicle shape and form	207
Fig. 16-1.	Adult dentition with quadrants for nomenclature	217
Fig. 16-2.	Adult upper right canine tooth showing internal structures	218
Fig. 16-3.	Normal and defective occlusion in the anterior teeth: (a) openbite, (b) normal bite, (c) overbite, (d) underjet, (e) normal edge to edge bite, (f) overjet	226
Fig. 16-4.	Upper first incisors showing various degrees of winging defects	227
Fig. 16-5.	Comparison of sphenoid bone with sacroiliac bones (anterior views)	228
Fig. 16-6.	Both scapulae (shoulder-blades) posterior view and placed beside each other	229
Fig. 16-7.	Course of prisms within tooth enamel showing sinusoidal arrangement: (a) single prism, (b) collection of prisms	235
Fig. 16-8.	Table of teeth/body correspondences	236-7

table of symbols

symbol	description
☉	Astrological glyph for the Sun
↓	Astrological glyph for Vulcan
☿	Astrological glyph for Mercury
♀	Astrological glyph for Venus
⊕	Astrological glyph for the Earth
☽	Astrological glyph for the Moon
♂	Astrological glyph for Mars
♃	Astrological glyph for Jupiter
♄	Astrological glyph for Saturn
♅	Astrological glyph for Uranus
♆	Astrological glyph for Neptune
♇	Astrological glyph for Pluto
⚷	Astrological glyph for Chiron
∞	Symbol for infinity and archangel Metatron
✡	Star of David, symbol for integration of spirit and matter

introduction

Humanity is fast approaching a crisis point in its evolution as it enters a new age of enlightenment. However the driving force for change is not some random mutation or alteration of the physical body during its existence on Earth. It has long been known amongst ancient religions and spiritual mystery schools the influence the spiritual realm has on earthly life. This is a book about Mercury within the fantastic journey that human souls have chosen to undergo through trial, tribulation and above all creative exploration on Earth. It is about Mercury in all its facets.

The book seeks to reveal the unified nature of Mercury as planet, mythic god, biological process and physical metal. It shows that there is no actual difference in the energy as between all these forms. A study of the spiritual perspective of early Earth cosmogenesis reveals the nature of Mercury as a primordial gas within the atmosphere of Earth. This gas was in effect the rays of energy radiating into the Earth from the newly formed planet as Mercury. However, long before the physical Mercury appeared, there was a process and a being of consciousness known as Mercury. The book attempts to portray the magic that underlies our world and Mercury's part in this. It is the first of a series of books exploring the influence of the solar system of planets within the Earth domain, through their metals and psychological influences.

Insightful study of the astronomy, astrology and mythology surrounding each planet reveals a profound correlation with the properties of the metal traditionally related to the planet in alchemical lore. The Sun relates to the metal Gold, the planet Mercury to the metal of the same name, Venus to the metal Copper, the Earth's Moon to Silver, Mars to Iron, Jupiter to Tin and Saturn to Lead.

The perspective here is on homoeopathic medicine, but the principles are applicable to many academic subjects of interest. The biological and toxicological properties of these metals throws further light on the classic picture within the materia medica of the homoeopathic remedy made from the metal. The power of homoeopathy, both for materia medica study and for finding the indicated remedy is always improved by greater understanding of the mechanism of action of the remedy. Hahnemann wrote of the vital energy as a basis of health, and that disease could only be understood by observing the dysfunction of this vital energy. I believe it is now time for homoeopathy to delve into this vital energy – to find the laws and principles that guide its behaviour. Such principles can only be found after acknowledging the existence of a supersensible spiritual realm, from which impulses stream and shape our world.

I hope a first reading of the book will provide much material for reflection. However some of the material requires an exercise of the faculties of imagination and meditation in order to grasp the subtle laws by which Mercury works. Another work - the 'Manual of Spiritual Healing', due for publication in 2003, will include some relevant techniques. However I trust Mercury itself will be able to guide the reader on this journey of discovery.

chapter 1

basic overview

Spiritual formation of the solar system planets

Mercury is the closest visible planet to the Sun, although there are planets even closer but as yet in etheric and astral form. Mercury developed out of the substance of the Sun soon after the separation of the Sun from the Earth during the early Old Sun phase of world history. The planets of our solar system are effectively the chakras or energy centres within the aura of the Sun.

Mercury vapour on Earth

Before the Sun had separated from the Earth (see p.40), the beings inhabiting the Earth/Sun were in an early primordial phase of the development of humanity. They were shadow beings with physical bodies made predominantly of warmth and fire/heat forces. The pulling away of the Sun allowed for the air element to manifest and interact with their fiery bodies, beginning the process of rhythmic breathing. As Mercury moved out of the Sun, its influence became energetically manifest on Earth. There is a spiritual law 'as above so below': everything that occurs in the material earthly realm has a spiritual counterpart, and vice versa. Thus the planetary energies of Mercury became manifest on Earth as gaseous Mercury vapours in the primordial Earth atmosphere. At any rate this atmosphere was very different to that present now, containing large quantities of sulphur, cyanide (carbon-nitrogen compounds) and gold (from the Sun's influence) amongst other toxic gases. The earthly beings could directly absorb and inhale these to provide sustenance. Solid physical ground did not exist and plant life lived in suspension within the atmosphere.

Through the cooling of the Earth, the Mercury vapour gradually condensed into liquid metal Mercury. In truth there is no energetic separation between the metal Mercury and the planet Mercury; they are one and the same consciousness; one and the same being. Later this being became depicted in myth as the god Mercury, also known as Hermes. Everything containing physical Mercury, or using Mercury processes in its physiology, can only be properly understood by this principle. Mercury is depicted as the messenger of the gods, linking the spiritual and material worlds, passing information back and forth between humanity and the gods. In effect Mercury not only carries, but also becomes the message. Mercury can thus incorporate blueprints from the divine worlds by integrating their substance and corporeality into the receiving physical structure.

Breathing process and astrality

The breathing process facilitates the integration of the spiritual with the human material realm. Mercury is the key vibration required by the primordial lungs to structure the alveoli. Indeed alveoli look very similar to drops of Mercury. Before the Mercury/Sun separation, the breathing process of the Earth inhabitant was unconscious, without actual air entry into or out of the physical structure. It would be more akin to surface diffusion of gases from the atmosphere through the outer 'skin' of the beings. The advent of Mercury enabled airway penetration of air into the being, into lung organs. The shift of consciousness this caused was profound. The astral body of human souls could now penetrate into the physical-etheric body unit. The astral body is that which perceives sensations, desires, feelings and emotions. It is the super-expanded and super-conscious extension of the lower emotional body that for many humans is still the seat of their conscious emotional life. When the much more multidimensional astral body is the centre for emotional life then the human can perceive sensations and feeling energy from great distances and from other time co-ordinates altogether. This enables experiences of déjà vu and sensing how others feel no matter where they are.

If the astral body were to not be able to penetrate the physical-etheric body then that person would not be aware of their emotions whilst living in physical awareness. They would have a very dim fish-like consciousness, barely awake and functioning on an unconscious level on Earth. The soul would reside in the spiritual realm and have a weak interaction with the lower embryonic collection of tissues. This is the consciousness of the embryo or foetus within the womb; it does not need to flow air into its lungs, which is instead full of fluid. All breathing is done for the embryo by the mother, who suffuses the required gases ready prepared through the placental blood. This recapitulates the old pre-Lemurian state of a very dim earthly consciousness, with a soft floating physical structure and an inability to breathe so as to aerate the physical body. At that time the human souls were being carried in the laps of higher spiritual beings in the spiritual plane.

Lemuria and the development of consciousness

Thus Mercury is vital to enable corporeality. This encapsulates the idea of the wakeful awareness of oneself as a soul-spiritual being on Earth. The person need not feel in tune with the spiritual realm. Rather, it is the conscious perception of oneself being on Earth, awake and with a sense of self.

Mercury governs the flow and incorporation of whatever blueprints are needed in other parts of the physical body. This connotes a prior state of separation having been induced in the physical body. Pre-Lemurian beings had an open and constant channel linking them to the spiritual realm whilst on Earth. The pineal gland at the vertex or top of their head provided a direct etheric link to the spiritual realm. This could be likened to a string controlling a puppet. These beings did not have eyes facing forwards and horizontally into the material world. They could not see the world they were in, but perceived themselves as beings in the spiritual world and with a channel of energy feeding into a body structure they could not consciously control in the material world.

This changed however in early Lemuria, after the Sun-Mercury separation, when the pineal gland descended into the developing brain – eventually becoming seated deep in the centre of the brain, slightly towards the rear where it is now. Initially a channel still connected this descending pineal gland with the top surface of the brain and head (there was no firm bony skull vault surrounding the brain as yet), which was called the 'parietal eye'. This eye eventually moved forwards (but sometimes backwards) to form the single horizontal eye of the Cyclops. When two eyes eventually developed, it enabled a binocular vision but also a stance of duality within the material world. Beings could no longer feel the same unity with the spiritual world or with spiritual beings. This recapitulates the breaking of the physical link between the foetus and mother when birth occurs and the umbilical cord is broken. In that ancient past this event was termed the fall of humanity. The separation from the spiritual realm really did occur, and earthly incarnated beings now felt a somewhat more independent existence from the spiritual realm.

Basic spiritual theme of the remedy

Metallic Mercury has been extensively used during the history of allopathic medicine (see p.139) and remains an important remedy in its homoeopathic form. In alchemy the planet and biological process of Mercury were utilised in subtle experiments to harness the vibration of the soul.

As a remedy the theme of Mercury generally concerns the communication of messages. As metal, Mercury is light and mobile, being liquid at room temperature. It is joyful and at ease with itself. That it easily coalesces rather than dissipating shows that it keeps the message intact yet flowing to its destination. It is able to aerate the whole organism, thus Mercury governs the breathing process. This includes the stoppage of breath in order to enter the spiritual world as in death processes, as well as enlivening breath processes.

The ultimate theme of Mercury is to allow the whole cosmos to interact with Earth citizens, to impart the myriad messages and communications that occur all the time from the spiritual world. Through Mercury communication skills are enhanced, and the throat chakra is further opened. It allows the soul to realise communication as a flow of multi-dimensional information. Awareness arises of Mercury's connections throughout the cosmos, yet it is very much able to bring this to material reality. Note Mercury's ability to bring heaven's messages from the gods to Earth and to the underworld. Upon looking back at oneself from the perspective of Mercury the soul can realise how much or little it communicates to those around itself. As this communication is increased by visualisation, the influence of Mercury can be greater, with a greater ability to translocate and flow consciousness into other worlds to disseminate knowledge therein.

chapter 2

homoeopathic picture

Fig. 2-1 lists the various Mercury remedies available in the materia medica. They have broadly similar indications.

Homoeopathic name	Chemical name
Mercurius vivus (Merc-viv)	Elemental Mercury Hg
Mercurius solubilis (Merc-sol)	Mercury oxide HgO
Mercurius dulcis (Merc-d)	Mercury (I) chloride Hg_2Cl_2 (calomel)
Mercurius corrosivus (Merc-c)	Mercury (II) chloride $HgCl_2$
Mercurius bromatum (Merc-br)	Mercury (II) bromide $HgBr_2$
Mercurius iodatus flavus (Merc-i-f)	Mercury (I) iodide Hg_2I_2
Mercurius iodatus ruber (Merc-i-r)	Mercury (II) iodide HgI_2
Mercurius aceticus (Merc-ac)	Mercury (II) acetate $Hg(CH_3.COO)_2$
Mercurius nitrosus (Merc-n)	Mercury (I) nitrate $Hg_2(NO3)_2$
Mercurius sulphide (Merc-s)	Mercury (II) sulphide HgS (vermilion)
Mercurius sulphuricus (Merc-sul)	Mercury (II) sulphate $HgSO_4$
Mercurius cyanatus (Merc-cy)	Mercury (II) thiocyanate $Hg(SCN)_2$
Mercurius oxycyanatus (Merc-ox-cy)	Mercury (II) oxycyanide $3Hg(CN)_2.HgO$

[Fig. 2.1]

Mercurius vivus is the name provided for the homoeopathic medicine derived from metallic Mercury, in elemental form. However, Samuel Hahnemann and other early homoeopaths considered the chemical compounds of Mercury to be most suitable for treating disease, since the elemental form was considered to have little dynamic action on human health. Eventually Hahnemann produced the black oxide of Mercury, known as Mercurius solubilis. This substance became the leading mercurial preparation throughout the homoeopathic world. However the toxicological symptoms of Mercurius vivus are often taken together with the proving picture of Mercurius solubilis in most materia medica. In this text, where the exact preparation is not shown (i.e. 'Mercurius') then the Merc-sol form is indicated.

The remedies are made in accordance with standard methodology in official homoeopathic pharmacopoeias – by a process of dilution and succession (shaking of the vial). Beyond a potency of 12c (a dilution factor of 10^{24}) there is, in theory, no longer any atoms left of the original metal Mercury or compound.

The pictures of the remedies that follow have been well described from the provings, clinical use and from the toxicological behaviour of the material substance.

Mercurius solubilis

Note that Mercurius vivus is practically the same as the picture in this form. The properties are as categorised:

Mentals
Seclusion and isolation
These are mentally introverted and emotionally withdrawn people. They are very nervous, timid, shy and are easily embarrassed in social situations, blushing easily. When approached or challenged, direct eye contact and conversation is avoided. There is extreme nervousness about being watched, including at work, this causing an inability to perform. If they feel watched they can feel a sudden depletion of muscle strength, tremor and muscle twitching and panic attack. They also have a deep need to obtain guidance from sources external to themselves, and have a deep insecurity as to the validity and strength of their own convictions.

Instability on all levels

They have very changeable moods and often change their mind. Routines are changed unpredictably. This can be beneficial because they easily adapt to their environment and are flexible, like a chameleon. They have the gift of the gab, have quick-witted speech and become comedians who think fast on their feet. However they may fall into a loss of personal identity through the excessive changeability. They then feel very isolated, without a sense of foundation, robotic like and anonymous - especially in the context of city life. They can be very difficult to pin down, and put up a front of a role other's want to see, such as method acting.

Deep internal emotional states of suspicion and negativity exist and they feel very different to others. This can lead to schizoid fragmented personality states. The personality can become extremely unstable and enter states of delusion and hallucination. Belief systems and role models lose their stable sense of foundation and the person no longer has a firm grasp of the present reality.

They try to cover up this inner state by appearing outwardly reserved and controlled. They have an emotional need for people to listen to them with undivided attention; otherwise they may feel very insecure.

There are strong inner impulses – such as to strike someone, but they try to suppress or hide these and appear outwardly calm. They do not know from where these impulses arise, but they seem to come from deep within their subconscious.

They may be revolutionary anarchists, either out of philosophical doctrine or from sheer impulse and restlessness.

Use of this remedy helps to clear fears of dying and illness. A sense of receptivity to the final outcome can be reached, and they come to feel in tune with their own inner feelings and impulses.

Restlessness and hurriedness
They cannot relax, but must be constantly on the go. They are especially restless at night and unable to sleep, yet also finding walking about intolerable - so that no position or activity gives them peace. They can have an irresistible desire to travel great distances and to far away places. They may hurry without thinking and so suffer the consequences of improper action.

Closed and detached
They can be very inconsiderate of others, and indifferent to everything in the world. They do not consider the consequences of their actions on others. (Note the poor adhesion of Mercury's metallic droplets to the surrounding surface.) Similarly they may not touch reality around them but appear very closed within themselves. If others attempt to get through this outer veil they may become suspicious, vulnerable and cautious. Indeed they may enter paranoid states of thinking everyone is their enemy.

Need for order amongst chaos
They feel everyone should know their place in society and that the public status quo should not be broken. They can become very conservative, needing a stable life to counterbalance their inner turmoil. This reflects the need for every micro-droplet of Mercury metal to be able to re-integrate into the whole again, and the god Mercury having the role to guide souls to their proper destination within the society of the spiritual realm. Note this is not at odds with the inherent instability and sense of anarchy they can exhibit as discussed above, for each soul has their unique picture of Mercury. They can have an inner conflict between this need for law and order and desire for anarchy.

Temperature
They are very sensitive to extremes of temperature, to heat and to cold. They can thus easily become chilled but also just as easily overheated. They may feel chilly in parts of their body whilst other parts feel normal or even hot. (Liken this to the properties of the metal Mercury within the thermometer.)

Sexuality
The Mercurius child can be sexually precocious, an early developer and sexually active from too early an age. This could manifest as early physical genital development and/or as flirtatious behaviour.

Breathing processes
This remedy improves the rhythmic flow of air by way of inhalation and exhalation and thus improves lung function. It aids the restructuring of physical lung tissue to enable improved respiration. Thus it can resolve scar tissue, chronic pus, lung cavitation, inflamed lung tissue or a structural loss of airway capacity in most other conditions. Many chronic lung states such as chronic bronchitis, emphysema, bronchiectasis, pneumonia (acute, recurrent or chronic), tuberculosis, fibrosing alveolitis, sarcoidosis and other restrictive and scarred lung diseases are amenable to vibrational Mercury treatment.

Inflammation
It clears pus and catarrh from the physical body by assisting the scavenging of pus by other white cells and preventing new pus formation. Note that pus is composed of dead white cells with dead and live microbes (for example, bacteria) in the fluid exudate.

There is a tendency in the patient to teeth decay, gum infections and throat infections. The tongue has an imprint of the teeth at its margins. The breath can be offensive; there is a metallic taste in the mouth and with excessive salivation. It helps chronic fatigue states especially when characterised by shortness of breath. There is a tendency to ear infections, such as otitis media.

Perspiration and discharges
They sweat heavily all over their body, and this can be an oily, foul smelling sweat that stains the bedclothes. They tend to have free secretions that may be thin, burning, foul or thick and purulent.

Anti-syphilitic
Mercurius solubilis is a major anti-syphilitic miasmatic remedy. Thus it clears auto-destructive body processes, especially when characterised by ulceration, necrosis or gangrene. This includes ulceration in the interior of the body, such as peptic or stomach/duodenal ulcers and ulcerative colitis.

It focuses especially on the heart, bone and nervous system with respect to the syphilitic miasm. There can be degenerative structural damage to these organs. Thus it treats cardiac valve defects (such as aortic valve stenosis, mitral valve regurgitation and so on), aortic aneurysm at thorax and abdominal levels, inflamed heart tissue such as endocarditis and myocarditis, and heart failure. Rather than functioning as a diuretic or pain relieving agent, its mode of operation is to help heart and blood vessel tissue to regenerate in accordance with normal healthy tissue blueprints.

As regards bone degeneration, there can be diseases such as osteoporosis, Paget's disease, deformed bony degeneration in crippling arthritis, bony spurs and bone tumours.

Any nervous system disease can be part of a Mercury picture, but commonly includes multiple sclerosis, cerebellar degeneration, peripheral neuropathy, strokes, Parkinson's disease, motor neurone disease and other spinal degenerative states, optic nerve degeneration and retinal diseases and auditory and vestibular balance nerve diseases such as Menieres disease. With nervous system degeneration there is a tendency to have tremor.

Mercurius corrosivus

Also known as Hydrargyrum bichloratum, this is Mercuric chloride. It is the elemental Mercury chemically bound with chlorine.

This remedy has a more severe and rapid action than Mercurius solubilis, and especially focuses on the gastrointestinal tract. All the symptoms of Mercurius solubilis will feature in this form. A common source for material toxicity is from amalgam fillings in the teeth, where the alkaline action of saliva on the Mercury leads to the chloride being formed. This is insidiously and continuously absorbed into the system, wreaking havoc, which may be irreparable.

Mentals
They can be more disconnected than usual, with wandering schizoid thoughts, great anxiety and mental instability.

Generals
There is a more intense generalised sweat, with chilliness especially worse in the open air. There is an insatiable thirst for cold drinks, with a constant dry mouth – although drinking may not relieve. There is an intense burning quality to most of the symptoms, especially at the throat, abdomen, rectum, and kidney region. Constrictive feelings exist in various body parts and discharges tend to be corrosive.

Particulars
There is an acute and ulcerative stomatitis, with red inflamed gums and soft palate of the mouth. Swallowing becomes almost impossible and can lead to retching and vomiting upon attempting to do so.

There can be loose and/or frequent diarrhoea, with a never-get-done or incomplete feeling of evacuation (tenesmus). Diarrhoea can be accompanied by violent burning and bleeding within the stool. Diseases matching such a picture include ulcerative colitis, typhoid fever and dysentery.

Mercurius iodatus flavus

This is the yellow Mercury iodide, also called Mercurous protoiodide. It is the elemental Mercury chemically bound with iodine. It is a strong yellow powder, without odour and tasteless. On exposure to light it rapidly decomposes. Historically it has been used as a medicament or ointment for the eyes.

Mentals
There is a feeling or delusion that a knife or blade is perforating their throat. Great fear and premonition of death accompanies this. A sense of others approaching them is felt, as if surrounded by enemies and about to be murdered. An impulse to kill may also arise, or other violent destructive feelings.

There is a strong desire to move, including travel. They can become quite manic, elated and hyperactive, perhaps constantly moving from place to place or from jobs.

They can have dreams of urinating.

Generals
There tends to be swollen glands, especially at the neck. Hot, cold and damp weather generally aggravates and they perspire easily. Discharges are common and often lumpy in character.

Complaints tend to be right-sided.

Particulars
Of note is a tendency to sore throats with thick tenacious mucus. The tongue can become thickly furred at its base with a yellow coat.

The elements of the periodic table
To understand the features of chemical and mineral based remedies within the homoeopathic materia medica, a study of the periodic table of elements is relevant. Furthermore the properties of the elements of the periodic table are meaningfully explained by an understanding of spiritual processes. Modern science attempts to understand the nature of an element from its physical properties and atomic structure. However a physical element is simply the most material manifestation of energy or a process.

The halogens are the group of elements including fluorine, chlorine, bromine and iodine. The essence of the halogen group can reveal a common theme to its Mercury compounds. The energetic theme of the halogens is to guide the integration of external and more collective ego consciousness into the sphere of the human individualised ego consciousness. Each human has a certain sense of self, which can be considered the current assemble of personality, soul and spirit combined into an ego or self. This imparts personal character and an ability to view the outside world as an individual separated from it. However, there are of course myriad ego consciousness units throughout the world, not being simply the rest of the human race but also the nature spirits, spirit guides, angels, planetary consciousness beings (such as Earth mother) and so on. The list of individuals in creation is infinite.

Through the halogens is imparted an appreciation of consciousness beyond the self. Thus iodine enables outside forces to stream into the personal consciousness and energy field, mostly through the portal of the personality and the throat chakra. In doing so it stimulates a process of integration by opening the head chakras and enabling the personality to let go of personal ego positioning (such as personal belief systems, goals and ambitions) and enter a state of transpersonal positioning (i.e. collective thinking and greater consideration of the whole picture). If this occurs prematurely, when the lower chakras and body cannot cope with the energetic activation, then a state of physical hyperactivity arises. Hyperthyroidism is the classical disease associated with the materia medica features of iodum (iodine). This condition is invariably associated with a blockage in the sacral chakra and adrenal glands, causing a poor earthly grounding of the new energy attempting to integrate into the personality at its throat chakra. There is also a blockage at the brow chakra and pituitary gland to do with poor inner perception of such energy.

The combination of Mercury with iodine can now be meaningfully understood. Mercury opens the aura and energy field up to the influence of iodine, especially at the throat chakra. Hence a gap appears at this region in the outer lining of the aura, enabling outside forces to stream in and provides a greater transpersonal awareness to the personality-soul unit. This explains the perception arrived at by many provers when they feel this etheric energy rift, as a sense of being stabbed in the throat and also a fearful quality of death. The death process is simply the awareness by the personality of its finite position as compared with the immortality of the spirit, and its having loosened the firm grasp it formerly had of the material realm as the only state of reality. Death is a portal of entry into the spiritual realm. If perceived whilst still 'alive' and present within a physical body it provides for a lifting of the veil of death and anchoring of the sense of immortality whilst still physically incarnate.

Mercurius iodatus ruber

This is the red mercuric iodide, or Mercury biiodide. It is a vivid red amorphous powder, stable below 127° C and without odour. It has been used as an antiseptic and disinfectant for inanimate objects.

Its features closely resemble Mercurius iodatus flavus, except that complaints generally tend to be right-sided, such as a right-sided sore throat, right-sided otitis and so on. The variation of the energetic theme is that this remedy has a greater flow of the subtle bodies into the physical-etheric body. In so doing the ego consciousness tends to flow along the right side of the body, anchoring through the liver into the metabolic activity of the body. The liver is where the warmth forces of the ego become immersed into the watery etheric organism of the body. Here the metabolism becomes stamped with the unique blueprint of the soul or ego so as to make the organic molecules individualised or personalised within the physical body. Each individual human has a unique metabolism (different rates of reactions, different nutrient substrate requirements, differences in metabolic end products and so on) and this is shaped by the personal biography of the soul and its multiple incarnations.

Mercurius oxycyanide

This is divalent Mercury (II) cyanide with Mercury (II) oxide. It is a new proving made in July 2002 meditatively as the source mineral material is too toxic to be produced by trituration (grinding with lactose using mortar and pestle). The actual compound is a class 6.1 poison, a severe marine and environmental pollutant and explodes on both impact and heat.

Single prover symptoms and case studies reveal the following effects:

Mentals
There is a sensation of foreboding, of doom and impending death. Fearful images can appear in the inner mind of demons, of ancient fiery elemental beings with enormous power. With this is a sensation of great strength in the arms and legs – especially in the hands and feet.

Particulars
It has a powerful effect on both lung and cellular respiration. There are severe suffocating sensations of breathlessness with constriction about the chest limiting lung expansion. It can consequently treat lung failure (from any cause, such as emphysema and chronic airways obstruction, pulmonary fibrosis and congestive cardiac failure with pulmonary odema).

It treats cyanotic diseases especially due to poisoning and blood disorders. These cause a deficiency in the oxygen carrying capacity of the blood. Examples of such poisons are carbon monoxide (such as from fire or combustion of fossilised fuel within a closed or unvented space), cyanide and lead – all of which severely disrupt the haemoglobin within the red blood cells. Patients will become severely de-oxygenated, with a bluish dusky skin colour. Sometimes there is coldness and a poor blood circulation, at other times there can be dilatation of blood vessels with a bounding blood circulation and heat flushes.

Spiritual theme of the remedy
The materia medica picture of this compound would be expected to observe the basic principles regarding the relationship between Mercury, oxygen and cyanide. The atmosphere at one time during ancient Earth contained Mercury compounds, cyanide and other gases, which would now be considered extreme poisons. The Earth at that time experienced the Old Saturn phase of evolution, whereby the fiery forces of ancient

Saturn were part of the matrix of Earth. The present Saturn of our solar system is a faint remnant of that once mighty planet. Saturn carries latent heat and fire that formerly existed within the Earth and also embodied by ancient elemental beings built of fire substance. The dragons and fiery salamanders of myth are but minor reflections of such beings. This remedy can awaken consciousness of this time on Earth.

In doing so, it activates deep memories within the collective psyche of humanity to do with the primordial past. The remedy can assist the soul that wishes to liberate from the time-line of reincarnation, karma and the burden of memory. The veil of death must be transversed for this to happen, hence the extreme death-like quality of the compound. That it relates more strongly to the lungs and breathing function than the metal Mercury alone in homoeopathic form is revealed by the additional elements of oxygen and cyanide. Oxygen is effectively a carrier for cosmic and spiritual sources of energy, inspired into the physical body with a degree of prana or vitality as well as objective alertness of the material world. Cyanide is an extreme cellular poison, lethal to most forms of biological life. In primordial Earth, however, it was far from poisonous – it was nutritive and invigorating to breathe into the physical form.

chapter 3

Mercury as metal

Metal and planet relationship

The metal Mercury present within our planet Earth bears more than a name resemblance to the planet Mercury. The ancients in their wisdom could perceive the relationships between the stellar bodies and various substances on Earth. When each planet was formed as a densification out of etheric vital substance and under spiritual laws, so also would the planet's essence appear in gaseous form on the primordial Earth. These were the original seven sacred metals and present as gases within the atmosphere. Thus Mercury existed once as a vapour on Earth, and became liquid as the Earth cooled over time.

Relationship with Old Saturn and lead

Mercury is unique amongst all the metals in being liquid at room temperature, yet remarkably it is almost twice as heavy as iron and fourteen x heavier than water. Thus it has retained some of its early nature, whereas the other metals already lost their gaseous and liquid nature far in the ancient past of Earth. Mercury in fact has a close relationship with Saturn for the purposes of conducting the ancient blueprints from Old Saturn through the modern version of Saturn and into the Earth. This is explained further in 'Homoeopathy of the Solar System: Saturn and Lead' within this series. Essentially the Old Saturn period in ancient Earth was a time of fire and heat forces only. Lead is the metal carrier of Saturn forces, and is a metal that carries latent heat. It behaves like a metal already near its melting point due to the Old Saturn fire and warmth forces held within its substance (even though it seems cold to physical touch). However the warmth of lead is not fresh and vibrant, but has energetically the quality at times of aged decay, or long-lived memories and sclerotic tendencies of habit. Such qualities can be cleared from the soul through the use of Saturn and its related homoeopathic lead (plumbum).

Mercury is responsible for enlivening and transforming the ancient forces held within Saturn and lead. Mercury can bring up deep ancient memories within the soul, such as from past lives, and yet make them seem to the soul as fresh and immediate as though that life were the present incarnation. Thus Mercury imparts a youthful quality to old ancient memories, and as a mythic God also appears young and vital. Similarly the metal Mercury is liquid, a sign that it has refused to age into a hardened solid form along with the ageing of the Earth, but chosen to retain the same youthful vigour of former days. As a liquid it appears bright, without losing its lustre though corrosion or rust formation. Conversely lead readily covers its lustre with a patina of lead oxide. Lead chooses to bury its old ancient memories of past lives under this veil of oxidation, whilst Mercury does not.

Mining of Mercury

The centre for metal Mercury mining is Europe, especially the mines of Almaden in Spain, active since ancient times. The quantities extracted from European mines far exceed that from the rest of the world. Different spiritual qualities are imbued in the different geographical zones of the planet. Thus Europe is the best conduit for the energy of the planet Mercury, and anchors this energy through its metal. European countries have the consciousness and culture able to sit comfortably in the present time frame and yet also retain a tradition of heritage and the past, with a vision for innovation and the future. In general, the New World, as depicted by the Americas and especially the USA, have the cultural quality of looking toward the future and escaping from humanity's past. Conversely, the Old World, as the Far East and Africa, have the cultural energy of holding to its roots and creeping into the future from the backdrop of deeply entrenched memories.

These are not simply wilful ideas of human society, but are actually different time frames programmed into our world by spirit to provide different evolutionary phases needed for souls to work with their biography over time. Each human soul is a unique biographical journey of multiple incarnations (not all having been on Earth) which are not strictly bound to linear space and time, but are better viewed as holographic experiences in a constantly changeable grid of space and time. The soul can step into any space and time co-ordinate it chooses to best provide the experiences it needs for that particular step of its journey. Overall Europe provides the proper foundation for the activity of Mercury – enabling Mercury to flow its energy into whatever past, present or future Earth reality is required of it, whether for the purposes of the individual soul journey or of planetary memory.

Cinnabar ore

The main ore of Mercury metal is cinnabar, which is the red sulphide of Mercury. This is a blende, in that Mercury has completely lost its metallic appearance in the compound (as opposed to a pyrite compound where a metal can still reveal itself through a metallic lustre). Sulphur has overcome the metallic nature of Mercury, and with it the sulphur has lost its ready volatility and tendency to become gaseous. Notably sulphur was also a major gaseous constituent of ancient primordial Earth, when the planet was much hotter than it is now due to the indwelling Sun forces still bound with the planet (the Sun had not yet separated from the ancient Earth). Sulphur carries the warmth forces of the soul into a relationship with the metabolic and etheric nature of the body. However it strives to return to its gaseous nature whenever possible. This explains the need for sulphur to escape from the decomposing physical body upon the exit of the soul; for it represents the movement of the soul's warmth and vitality forces out of its former physical nature. Cinnabar is an intense scarlet colour, of value to the painter, and practically the most energetic red colour possible within the visible light spectrum.

To understand the spiritual nature of cinnabar requires an appreciation of the vibrational qualities of both Mercury and sulphur as gases. As discussed later in this section, Mercury gas is readily able to flow into the myriad alternate and parallel realities of soul existence within the world, and provides information to whatever soul aspect requires it. Through knowledge comes power to overcome limitation. Sulphur gas on the other hand conveys the spiritual warmth of love and fiery zeal of drive from the soul into the Earth reality it seeks to express through. During evolution, human souls have entered karmic agreements with other human souls to accept limitation, oppression and duality based power struggles as a mirroring process for the internal separation from one's true mastery as a spiritual being. Such binds literally trap souls in an alternate reality that has been called hell. This is actually a human subconscious construct, or holographic virtual reality for experiencing the consequences of impurity of the soul. It is sulphur and its fumes that are needed to anchor the soul's warmth forces in this realm, and in so doing the sulphur becomes tainted with foul and dense energy. Through the chemical bind with Mercury as cinnabar, the sulphur has led the forces of Mercury into this underworld realm of the human mind and soul. This is symbolised by the journey of the god Mercury in leading the souls who have just 'died' to their next destination, including to Hades the underworld. The passionate red colour of cinnabar reveals the fiery forces active in this subterranean realm, which are required to cleanse and purify the souls therein.

The karmic memories that a soul carries are in part stored in the vital energy of the blood. In further incarnations the soul retains these karmic cords with other souls by way of blood ties and problematic cell receptor groupings. The groups which medical science understands are based on the various surface receptors on the red blood cell membranes, such as the ABO groups, Rhesus and so on. However this is only the material view of the history and influence of blood groups and with respect to its mixing between people. Blood carries ties on energetic levels that have yet to be discovered by medical science and which link souls to each other. These bonds are present on multiple levels such as family relationships, tribal, national, religious and various soul groupings.

Properties of liquid Mercury

At room temperature it is liquid, and only solidifies at -39° C. It is very conductive to electricity and heat when solid, as well as very malleable and ductile (can be stretched to a fine wire). As a pure liquid it does not tarnish on ordinary exposure to atmospheric oxygen, but when heated to near boiling point it oxidises to Mercuric oxide. Otherwise liquid Mercury is stable in air and water and does not react to most acids and alkalis. It is the heaviest of all known liquids, being 13.6 x heavier than the equivalent volume of water. It can even float stone, iron and lead on its surface. This liquid state is reflective of Mercury retaining its youthful state. It has more or less the same quality as it had during the early Earth period, when all metals were once liquid and the Earth was warmer. Earlier still on Earth, the metals were gaseous, and Mercury still retains an easy ability to vaporise, at only 359° C. A spilt drop of Mercury can soon disperse to fill the whole room with its vapour. In fact many of the qualities of Mercury (planetary and metal) could best be understood when perceiving its gaseous nature. In this form it is very sensitive to the realm of thought and information, at higher dimensions such as the fifth (which is the dimension of reality for thought-form activity). This is required of Mercury to fulfil its role of bringing messages from the spiritual and cosmic realms into the earthly material and underworld realms. Mercury must therefore be able to travel throughout the vibrational spectrum of density very easily and lightly. Mercury gas is literally able to communicate to the unseen spiritual beings at higher dimensions of reality. Upon liquefaction it retains this message. In a sense metallic Mercury behaves like a conscious being with the ability to live and breathe.

A quote from the commentary of Theodore Kerkringiusin in the Latin version of the great alchemical work of Basil Valentine 'Currus Triumphalis Antimonii' is of relevance by way of illustration:

'Let me tell you then that all metals and minerals grow in the same way from the same root, and that thus all metals have a common origin. This first principle is a mere vapour extracted from the elementary earth through the heavenly planets and, as it were, divided by the hot sidereal distillation of the Macrocosmos. This sidereal hot infusion, descending from on high into those things which are below, with the aero-sulphurous property, so acts and works as to engraft on them in a spiritual and invisible manner a certain strength and virtue. This vapour afterwards resolves itself in the earth into a kind of water, and out of this mineral water all metals are generated and perfected. The mineral vapour becomes this or that metal according as one or the other of the three first principles predominates, i.e., according as they have much or little mercury, sulphur, or salt, or an unequal mixture or their weights. Hence some metals are fixed; some are permanent and unchangeable; some are volatile and variable, as you may see in gold, silver, copper, iron, tin, and lead. Besides these metals, other minerals are generated from these three principles; according to the proportion of the ingredients, we have vitriol, antimony, marcasite, electrum, and many other minerals.'

In future Earth, Mercury will become solid at ambient temperature. This will be a great time of exteriorisation of the spiritual hierarchy and manifestation of heaven on Earth. The spiritual realm will be as 'real' and solid to the physical senses as the material realm is now, and the lines of communication governed by Mercury between these realms will be perceived as solid pathways or information highways.

Mercury easily retains its shape of the drop. It also easily disperses into multiple tiny droplets at the slightest jolt with each fragment as round as the original drop. Its cohesive tendency is so great however that these soon join together again. Its common name, qicksilver, stems from this property. Yet despite this it does not moisten the surface it rests upon and with this poor adhesion is able to flow very quickly and easily without leaving a trace. This reveals Mercury's nature to carry a signal or message without distortion. Like a truly reliable messenger, it does not alter the information it carries from one realm to another. It can enter realms and travel vibrationally into any of the many mansions of this world (alternate and parallel realities, of which there are a vast number on, around and inside Earth) without losing its essential good nature.

Mercury the god is depicted as a great diplomat who can enter any situation and win over others with his fine wit and playfulness.

These properties differ when mixed with other metals, and then Mercury can dissolve other metals to form amalgams and solutions. It behaves to metals rather like water to mineral salts. The metals particularly able to dissolve into Mercury are the softer metals, such as silver, gold, copper and tin. Iron and aluminium resist solubility and thus can be used in flasks to carry Mercury. All these metals are aligned to the other sacred planets of the solar system. However it is only Mars and the Earth which can function somewhat independent of Mercury with respect to receiving messages form the wider cosmos. The other 'planets', Saturn, Jupiter, Venus, the Sun and the Moon all require to interact with Mercury in order to receive their cosmic signals. Mars can and does act to receive signals from the cosmos outside of the sphere of Mercury, and possesses a degree of assertiveness, sense of adventure and courage that the other planets therefore lack. Similarly Earth can receive messages directly from the cosmos outside of Mercury's influence. Since iron is the metal for Mars and aluminium relates to the Earth, these two metals can resist the dissolving action of Mercury.

Properties of Mercury light

A Mercury vapour lamp, containing Mercury gas within the light bulb, radiates a peculiar blue-green light. A human lit by this light will appear like a corpse, without the healthy reddish pink glow of the skin. Also the light is strongly chemically catalytic, triggering chemical changes in many organic liquids. The liquid state is where metabolic reactions can properly find their place, and the naturally liquid state of Mercury is well suited to mediate here.

Light is an energy that can travel deep into material substance, to the point of becoming invisible to the naked eye and yet still present. Thus light is present within the cells and the seemingly dark core of the human body. It is especially active as light carrying phosphate within adenosine triphosphate (ATP) molecules in the cells. ATP is the 'energy packet' providing quick energy to drive various cell functions, including secretory (such as gland cells), motor (muscle cells) or electrical (nerve cells). The phosphate present within ATP is charged with light, which itself has been released from carbohydrate (sugar) metabolic breakdown. Sugar is a store of light originally harnessed from the Sun by plants. Animal and human cells reverse the plant process of photosynthesis to utilise this stored light.

Light also descends deep into the Earth crust and core. Indeed there is nowhere in creation where light cannot flow, even if it appears dim or darkened. Mercury light has a special quality of penetrating deeply into material substance and even deeper into suppressed subconscious arenas of the human psyche and the subterranean realms of Earth. In so doing Mercury is fulfilling its role of descending into the underworlds, and of guiding souls into the dark realms of shadow between lives when such a journey is required. Thus its light gives the appearance to a living being as if dead and a corpse, for its light shines on the path followed by this soul after it leaves the physical body at death.

Mercury and the atmosphere

Mercury has had a profound influence on the atmospheric oxygenation of planet Earth. Without gaseous Mercury within the early Earth atmosphere it would not have been possible to form oxygen and thus sustain biological life as we now know it. In its liquid state at normal room temperature it is impervious to the effects of damp and oxygen. It does not rust, unlike the easy corrosion of iron. Iron is more completely incarnated into the material realm than Mercury and has allowed itself to be a carrier for oxygen through the rust transformation.

However Mercury appears to inhale oxygen upon being heated, as if sucking it in from the atmosphere around it. Further heating then causes Mercury to release this oxygen, this forming the basis of industrial oxygen extraction. It was also the means by which oxygen was initially discovered. In a sense Mercury behaves like a metallic lung, and this breathing cycle is anchored into the human lungs under the influence of vibrational Mercury.

HOMOEOPATHY OF THE SOLAR SYSTEM: MERCURY

In primordial Earth prior to Old Sun, before the Sun had actually separated from Earth, there was an absence of a real atmosphere. From the perspective of multidimensional reality, the atmosphere represents the forces active upon the Earth from distant planetary and star systems. The atmosphere is literally interpenetrated by such channelled energies, and thus provides the basis for the higher dimensions to eventually manifest in material form. The fourth-dimension or astral plane has a flow consciousness, rather like the dream state. Thus the fourth-dimensional influence on the Earth atmosphere is the actual basis to the flow of energy (such as radio waves, microwaves, infra-red, gravitational waves, electrical fluxes) and of objects (such aeroplanes, birds, microbial particles, insects and so on). It is not mechanical force that propels and causes flight of objects in the atmosphere, but astral force.

The fifth-dimension is a mental plane holding thought-forms, and these are beyond the limitations of space and time. In effect all thought and knowledge is accessible from anywhere and from any time by tuning into the fifth-dimension. The influence this has when incorporated into the Earth atmosphere is to provide the proper energetic scaffolding for the array of information held within it and transiting through it. At any one time there is an immense amount of information coursing through the atmosphere. Human-made examples are satellite, radio and telephone communications. From nature, the sounds of wind, birdsong, insect noises, dolphins, whales and the many sounds from mammals (wolves, dogs, cows, sheep to name but a few) are all responsible for stabilising the matrix of energy or the information database which is the natural world. Many signals stream through the atmosphere from the wider cosmos, carrying zillions of messages for Earth and humanity.

When the Sun separated from the Earth at Old Sun, the atmosphere was as yet full of fumes which would be toxic to life now, including methane and cyanide gases. There was negligible oxygen. Mercury forming from the body of the Sun at a later date brought about the presence of Mercury gas in the Earth atmosphere, this metal being the vibration of the planet manifest in the microcosm of Earth. Since the Earth was still very hot, the Mercury gas functioned as a breathing organism for the Earth atmosphere, thus sucking into itself the pranic energy from distant planets and stars and then releasing this into the Earth atmosphere in the form of oxygen. This was the inhalation and exhalation activity respectively of Mercury.

Chemical catalytic properties

Mercury in ionic form reacts with other substances in two valences or electrical charges. The ionic forms of Mercury, which are active within the fluid sphere, were developed after the Moon separation from Earth, in Old Moon. In this period Earth underwent development of the water element and the realm of subconsciousness. The initial valency formed was the univalent mercurial form, by which it binds to other elements as a single positively charged moiety, giving away one of its negatively charged electrons in its outer atomic shell. A typical compound thus formed is horn ore, also known as calomel, which is a light-sensitive insoluble Mercury chloride, that has to be artificially produced nowadays as it is rare in nature. Its properties are very similar to silver, with which it is related in that silver formed on Earth at the initial Moon separation alongside the univalent Mercury.

The Moon had to separate from Earth otherwise earthly surface inhabitants would be forever dependent on the rich nurturing energy provided by the Moon as within the Earth. Humans were fed directly by the Earth-Moon combination through etheric umbilical cords connecting their physical bodies to the joint planetary body. The physical bodies of these early humans were soft, rounded and without a solid skeleton. Their blood was coloured white, being without red blood cells due to the lack of iron in material manifestation (Mars not yet projecting its energy onto the planet). The lack of iron in the blood caused a lack of expression of free will and egocentricity. Since the Moon's energy represents the past and foundational memory, then the pulling away of the Moon caused a tearing away of the very sense of foundation and of the memory of their past away from the human inhabitants. The Earth lost its sense of past planetary memory, which instead became stored in etheric devices under the separated lunar surface. The Moon at that early phase of separation still had a vitalised and warm energy. Over a long period of time, the subconscious realm of Earth and of humanity came to a rigid and dense state of petrified memories, unresolved emotional attachments and unrequited issues of all sorts. This has caused the rigidification of the present Moon into the dense cratered body it is now.

The bivalent form of Mercury came into being at this later time, after the Moon had started to mummify and harden into its current corpse-like state. In the bivalent form, Mercury forms corrosive compounds of Mercury chloride which is the Mercurius corrosivus of the materia medica.

Mercury chemically reacts directly with carbon to form organic compounds, such as Mercury trioxy-acetic acid. In such states it binds avidly to organic biological tissue and can thus accumulate for long periods and at toxic levels without being excreted in appreciable amounts.

Chapter 4

Toxic effects of Mercury poisoning

Forms and uses of Mercury

Mercury exists in three forms; as an element, as an inorganic ion (with one or two positive charges), and organic compounds such as CH_3Hg^+. The absorption and toxicity varies amongst these different forms. Sources of elemental and inorganic Mercury poisoning are usually accidents from heating Mercury in a closed space. This includes improper use of scientific apparatus, electrical equipment, dental amalgams, feltmaking, disinfectants, preservatives and button (disc) batteries. Sludge collected from electrical batteries was recycled to reclaim the Mercury therein, but considerable quantities of sludge have found their way into landfills and discharge into waterways. Much of this has accumulated in rivers and lakes, causing widespread damage to waterlife. The battery industry has converted to safer types recently, such as diaphragm cells. Environmental health enforcement has overall reduced the spillage and dumping of Mercury.

Some newborn babies have absorbed Mercury from accidental damage to the elemental Mercury switches in their incubators. Another major source of Mercury within the environment is the natural degassing of the earth's crust, including terrestrial landmass, rivers and oceans. Part of this is from fossil fuel, which may contain up to 1ppm (parts per million) of Mercury. About five thousand tonnes of Mercury is overall released from the burning of coal, gas and petroleum products. Other sources are from steel and iron plants, crematoriums and refuse incineration.

Metallic or elemental Mercury is present either as a liquid or as gas. It has a small degree of water solubility and somewhat greater lipid solubility. Inorganic Mercury exists as Mercuric salts Hg^{2+} and Mercurous salts Hg^+. The former is much more water-soluble and toxic in its compounds than the latter ionised form. The least water-soluble form is cinnabar (see p.20), which is its natural ore, HgS.

Organic Mercury compounds contain covalent bonds with carbon. The usual forms are alkylmercurials (methyl- and ethylmercury), arylmercurials (phenylmercury) and a family of alkoxyalkyl Mercury diuretics. Organic forms tend to react easily with inorganic and other organic forms, cross biological membranes easily and are usually lipid soluble. The most important toxicological difference between the various organic forms is their degree of degradation within the body, some break down more readily. Sources of organic Mercury are largely due to the burning of coal and other fossil fuels. Mining, smelting and refining processes also contribute. Most organic Mercury eventually reaches the sea and becomes concentrated in sea creatures, especially in predators such as seals and whales. Various poisoning epidemics have occurred from methyl Mercury contamination within ingested fish and shellfish.

Some organic methyl Mercury toxicity has occurred from fungicides leaching into crop seeds. These are mostly the alkylmercury compounds. Scientific analysis has measured over twelve thousand microbes usually found in or on crop seeds. These would reduce the chances of germination and proper plant growth, and Mercury-based fungicides were very popular during the 1960s. However large-scale poisoning of whole communities occurred through this action and organic Mercury compounds continue to enter the food chain today. The use of Mercury fungicides has now generally been banned.

Mercury bichloride solution was formerly used as a lavage (washing out) solution to destroy cancer cells that had metastasised or spread throughout the abdominal cavity. This points to the ability of Mercury to inhibit excessive independent life of the cell within the organism (see p.148). Thus Mercury has been used for some time to kill cancer cells and microbes whether in the human body or in the environment, but with long term toxic effects.

Absorption of Mercury

Mercury in elemental form is mostly absorbed through inhalation into the lungs. Hardly any enters through the gastrointestinal tract. Inorganic Mercury can be relatively easily absorbed orally through the gut, the skin and by inhalation. Organic Mercury also generally enters orally through the gut but much less often by inhalation and hardly at all by skin absorption.

Distribution of Mercury after absorption

Elemental Mercury is very fat-soluble and is also converted to the inorganic form within the blood. It crosses the blood brain barrier (which is a tight junction between blood vessel cells and the surrounding brain to limit drug and toxins from normally crossing into the brain) and becomes trapped in brain tissue. It can cross the placenta to affect the foetus. It also deposits in the kidneys, liver and heart. Inorganic Mercury mostly concentrates in the kidneys, and hardly crosses the blood brain barrier. Organic Mercury varies in its distribution depending on the exact organic structure, such as alkyl or methyl groups. Generally they are easily fat-soluble and cross the blood brain barrier and placenta. Some types therefore distribute throughout the body.

Toxic effects

Kidney damage, leading to renal failure tends to occur with inorganic Mercury but rarely from elemental or organic forms, even though these can also deposit in these organs. However elemental and organic forms tend to damage the blood brain barrier and lead to brain damage. Any part of the brain, spinal cord and peripheral nervous system can be affected, reminiscent of syphilitic infection (which also damages the nervous system, see p.153).

The inorganic form can cause severe necrosis and ulceration of the gut wall, leading to profuse bleeding and diarrhoea.

Lung damage tends to occur from elemental Mercury inhalation. Inflammation occurs within the airways and alveoli to cause exudate and oedema (fluid accumulation). Severe breathlessness occurs from blockage of airways through the shedding of inner airway linings. Lung sheaths (pleural membranes) and airway walls can rupture. In the long term the lungs can become scarred, with fibrosis, chronic pleural effusions (fluid layers around the lungs) and bronchiectasis (abnormally dilated airways with wasted air space causing inefficient ventilation).

Symptoms of toxic poisoning

Elemental Mercury usually causes symptoms of acute toxic exposure after inhalation of Mercury vapour. There can be an initial fever, chills, shortness of breath and headache within several hours. Later there are abdominal cramps and diarrhoea and reduced vision. Severe cases lead to lung failure, pneumothorax (ruptured lung tissue) and death. Sometimes fits, renal failure and liver damage occur. On the other hand chronic poisoning usually occurs in the workplace, such as dental offices. The usual symptoms are mouth symptoms (gingivitis or gum inflammation, increased salivation, mouth ulcers), tremor and psychological changes. These include insomnia, loss of appetite, shyness, emotional lability (mood swings) and memory loss. Nerve damage can cause motor or sensory weakness.

Acute poisoning with inorganic Mercury causes symptoms of a burning mouth, sore throat, nausea, vomiting, gingivitis, mouth ulcers and oesophageal ulceration. Furthermore abdominal pain, weakness, fatigue, pallor, bleeding in the gut with vomiting blood, shock and collapse can occur. Acute renal failure can occur. In chronic inorganic Mercury poisoning the symptoms are usually similar to the situation of chronic poisoning by elemental Mercury.

Organic Mercury poisoning can display symptoms similar to that of inorganic Mercury. Additionally there tends to be more physical nervous system damage, causing sensory neuropathy with numbness, tingling and incoordination. Other common features include spastic contractions of muscles, hyperactive reflexes, tremor, visual defects, hearing damage, poor concentration and emotional lability.

Of note is the great variability in humans for susceptibility to Mercury toxicity, which contributed to the blasé attitude amongst many early medical physicians who believed Mercury to be safe medicinally. Some people have been noted to absorb large quantities of Mercury without any seeming untoward effects. Others have suffered terribly from much smaller quantities. The toxic effects of Mercury however clearly match the classic homoeopathic picture which stems from the law of similars.

Chapter 5

Cosmological principles

Septenary division of all bodies

The soul of the solar system is a vast being known as the solar logos and called Helios. All planets within the solar system and life forms thereon are within and part of this great being, including humanity. Each planet in effect represents a chakra or centre of energy within the solar logos. However the physical planet that is visible is only a small part, the densest material manifestation of the solar chakra that it represents.

Each planet is part of its own individual scheme of evolution of which there are a total of ten. The entire solar system evolves as each planetary scheme unfolds through the incarnation and progressive experience of monads (individual soul-spiritual units) within them (Fig. 5-1). The solar logos turns its attention to each of the ten at a time, thereby accelerating the evolution of life forms within that particular scheme. Its current focus is on the Earth scheme, which is the third in the series overall. The lesson of evolution varies within each scheme and that of Earth is the need to surrender the lower self or personality to the higher self of soul-spirit. The particular qualities addressed through the Earth process are sacrifice, the courage to overcome fear and the need to transmute personal pain and suffering.

All objects in the spiritual as well as the material realms have a septenary or seven-fold structure. There are seven globes or chains within each planetary scheme (Fig. 5-2). In other words there are six companion chains to the physical chain existing, thus Earth has six other chains of Earth as part of its seven-fold makeup. The evolution of life proceeds from the first to the seventh chain. Furthermore within

COSMOLOGICAL PRINCIPLES

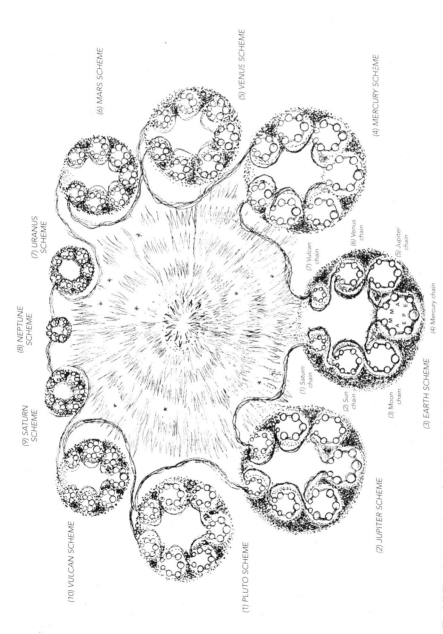

[**Fig. 5.1**] *The ten planetary schemes of evolution within the solar system, each supporting spiritual beings during their incarnations. The Earth scheme is the third in the series overall. There are seven globes or chains within each planetary scheme. M – mental, A – astral, E – etheric, P – physical are the primary level of focus within the chain.*

each chain there are seven rounds or cycles along which the impulse of evolution proceeds, from the first to the seventh round. At the end of each round there is a transfer of energy to the next round within the series, the former round entering a period of rest. At the last seventh round, there will be a transfer of energy to the next planetary chain, therefore all seven rounds of the former chain must die or extinguish.

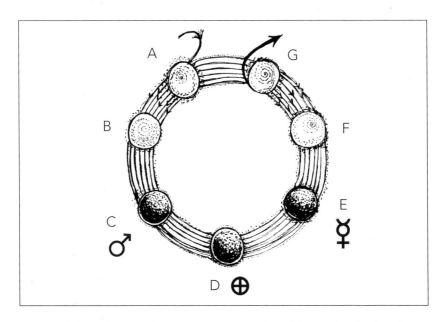

[Fig. 5.2] *Earth chain with seven rounds. Stages A to D represent involution of the spiritual impulse, descending into matter. Stages D to G represent the evolution of matter, returning to pure spirit. Earth is presently nearing the end of phase D. Mercury governs the evolution of Earth in the next phase E.*

The first three rounds of a planetary chain are formative and consolidating in nature, when the planet and its inhabitants are becoming materialised out of original fiery-mist. The first round of the Earth scheme is known as Old Saturn, the second round called Old Sun (when the Sun separated properly from Earth) and the third known as Old Moon (when the Moon separated from the Earth). It is during the fourth round that true solidification and materialisation occurs. The last three rounds then focus on returning to a state of spirit, with progressive etherealisation of matter to universal fiery-mist again. Earth is presently in her fourth round and in the fourth chain of evolution within the third planetary scheme. This represents an immeasurable length of time, incomprehensible to the human mind. Within the present chain there have been three previous rounds and there are three yet to come, when humans will assume their God and co-creator status again. Great sages and spiritual leaders over the last several thousands of years have developed the qualities of the future fifth and sixth rounds of Earth, whilst incarnating in the current fourth round. The powers of these great beings are equivalent to those of the average human in these future rounds. Additionally, within each Earth round there is a further septenary division into seven root races of humanity (see p.186 for discussion of reproductive patterns of the root races).

The other visible planets of our solar system are not actually the other planets within the Earth scheme of seven chains and rounds. Rather they are the visible materialised globes of their own planetary chains. Each planet is part of a septenary unit, their upper chains as invisible as the other Earth chains are to present humanity. Mercury is far older than the Earth, and in a much later stage of evolution with respect to its own planetary chain. Nonetheless these other planets impart their peculiar influence on the course of evolution on Earth. The overall rulership of each chain within the Earth planetary scheme is shown on the diagram. The Moon is particularly influential, having been the recent influence for the third chain and very formative to the fourth chain. Mercury is the overall guide for the present fourth chain, exerting a powerful influence on all earthly affairs until the shift to the fifth chain.

The visibility of the other solar system planets known by science is due to their adaptation to the peculiar vibration of the human race at this time. Humans can currently see Mercury, Venus, Mars, the Moon, Jupiter, Saturn, Uranus, Neptune and Pluto because of their direct material role in human affairs. Inhabitants of these other planets can respectively see our own Earth and perceive humans, and they also have their own chain of evolution to undergo.

Nebulae theory of the solar system

A nebula is a state of elemental and basic substance in dissociation, often seen spiral shaped. However it is more than simply gaseous – but is self-luminous and contains energy and spiritual vibrations which science cannot measure. Science hypothesises that the planets were all detached from the Sun, and that they were all once of one substance. This suggests the initially more or less homogenous and diffuse matter of the nebula became concentrated and condensed under forces of mass and gravity into the spherical planets existing now. The theory claims that the gaseous (and perhaps partially liquid) constituents of this nebula assumed the shape of a thin disc and underwent rotary motion. The centrifugal forces then overcame the cohesive powers holding it together, causing huge rings of substance to detach from the outer margins. These detachments then condensed under their own gravitational weight into the planets, and continued their orbit around the centre, in the same plane as each other, rotating on their axis as they orbited. Mechanical principles presumed that the inner bodies should be rotating much faster than those bodies further outward. Also that the more dense bodies should be thrown off last, for greater centrifugal force is needed to overcome their gravitational cohesion to the central Sun. Finally the nebulae theory holds that the satellites (moons) of the planets formed either from material thrown off from their own substance, or captured external detritus under their gravitational pull.

Ancient astronomers, however, often spoke of planets and stars forming out of the etheric substance of the universe, rather than on mechanical and material principles. There are divine builders, or great spiritual beings, that oversee such formations. Blueprints are required and intelligence is part of the grand design. The universe is full of intelligent consciousness beings, which play their part in creative, life giving and destructive processes of stellar and planetary bodies.

There are far too many discrepancies in the scientific nebulae theory for it to make sense, some of which are listed overleaf:

- Although it is closer to the Sun, Venus is less dense than Earth – a mechanical pulling away in accordance with graduations of density should make Venus situate further away. Similarly Uranus is denser than Saturn, but is further away from the Sun, again defeating the idea of centrifugal pull.

- The planets have many variations in the inclination of their rotational axis and even their orbits do not agree with the sense of a central origin.

- The planets have too great a variation in their relative sizes to apply to a central origin of mass.

- The meteors and comets working through the solar system are not convincingly explained as residue of the original nebulae.

- The satellites of Jupiter are 288 times denser than the main planet, which defeats any claim of their originating from its main substance.

- The satellites of Neptune and Uranus have a retrograde (reversibly oriented) motion, which would be difficult to explain if these satellites are simply mechanical creations of the main body or even captured satellites.

- The rotation of Mercury about its axis is approximately one-third that of Earth and its density is only about one-quarter greater than Earth. However these values are not enough to explain why its polar compression is more than ten times greater than that of Earth.

- Jupiter has an equatorial rotation about its axis twenty seven times greater than Earth, and is one-fifth the density of Earth. However its polar compression is seventeen times greater than that of Earth, and again cannot be explained by these values.

- Saturn has an equatorial velocity about its axis fifty five times greater than Mercury, which would have required a proportionally greater centrifugal velocity for Saturn. However its polar compression is only three times greater than Mercury, which also cannot be mechanically explained.

- Even more inexplicable is why the Sun has no significant polar compression or bulging at its equatorial region, suggesting the lack of the same centrifugal forces that had presumably led to the creation of the planets.

Spiritual science would otherwise teach that the bodies of the solar system are imbued with intelligence and the existence of many laws, energetic causes and effects as part of its grand design.

Formation of Mercury after Old Sun separation from Earth

In spiritual cosmological history, the planets were formed out of spiritual events and under the guidance of spiritual beings. Humanity instead seeks to understand the formation of the planets from some sort of mechanical grouping of substance under the influence of poorly understood forces such as gravity. Modern science presumes that at first instance the Sun formed and the planets developed as various foci of density in circulation around it, the furthest planets forming before those nearest the Sun. However there were many cycles of evolution preceding our present cycle and we are currently in the fourth great round of Earth evolution (see p.36). At the beginning of this fourth round, the Earth still contained within it the substance of the Sun, the Moon and the inferior planets (Mercury and Venus).

The time came when density prevented the solar beings within Earth from being able to fulfil their purpose. The Sun separated from the Earth and was at that stage still much larger than the present Sun. The Earth then underwent a tremendous coarsening. The Sun meanwhile separated out of its being the planets Mercury and Venus. Planets that are nearer to the Sun from the perspective of Earth are called inferior. Those planets further away from the Sun than the Earth are known as superior planets. The inferior planets, with the Earth and Moon, represent inversions of the cosmic energy streaming into our solar system and channel these impulses into inner realities. The superior planets of Saturn, Jupiter and Mars directly receive cosmic impulses and express these in the outer planes of reality. The inferior planets are related to the superior planets in a polar fashion. Thus Mercury is the inverse of the energy of Saturn. Venus is the inverse of the energy of Jupiter. Earth with Moon are together the inverse of the energy of Mars.

However the ancient astronomers and spiritual leaders also altered the naming of the planets Mercury and Venus, so as to reverse their characters. Thus Mercury was altered to incorporate some of the characteristics of Venus and Venus altered to incorporate some of the characteristics of Mercury. This can appear confusing to modern spiritual scientific thinkers but over time will become intuitively apparent.

Mercury is chiefly connected with the Spirits of Personality, also called the 'Archai'. The Archai are a race of beings who achieved self-realisation through deep awareness and reliving of their past. For this purpose they were required to live within and through the warmth bodies of the beings from Old Saturn. Old Saturn, as recapitulated by the present Saturn, was the initial holding bay for the fire spirits from the spiritual cosmos to enter and take hold of life within our solar system. The initial stage of material incarnation in the solar system was the presence of fire and warmth forces only. The bodies of the Old Saturn beings were composed only of differing degrees and qualities of warmth and fire. This imparted to them the qualities of zeal, life purpose and destiny. The Archai, by entering these ancient states of warmth and living through them, awakened themselves to the life purpose of these primordial spiritual beings desiring to incarnate into our solar system. Mercury was the planetary backdrop for the Archai to manifest the Old Saturn energies in a creative and new way.

Chapter 6

Mercury's astronomical properties

Orbit and rotation

Orbit around the Sun
Mercury is the closest known physical third-dimensional planet to the Sun. It orbits the Sun in eighty eight (87.97 precisely) days; this is the sidereal orbit (as considered objectively from the cosmic viewpoint). During one sidereal revolution a planet moves through the zodiac once to return to its starting point. From the perspective of the Earth it can never be more than 28° away from the Sun, thus hardly appearing as an independent object from the Sun.

Mercury is an inferior planet, which indicates it is closer than Earth to the Sun. It thus appears to oscillate to the left and right of the Sun over the course of its orbit, and it will only become visible during these periods (Fig. 6-1). Visibility also requires the Sun to be below the horizon, for its glare masks the light of Mercury. It will become invisible when closer (from the Earth's perspective) to the Sun. Mercury is seen as a morning planet in the east and an evening planet in the west (Fig. 6-2). Additionally, the sunset and sunrise moves slightly along the horizon over the course of the year. The movement of Mercury similarly must shift laterally to follow that of the Sun. It also changes the angle of movement due to variation in the angle of the ecliptic (the apparent path of the Sun and planets around the Earth over the year). The position of Mercury above the horizon at east or west is therefore a combination of its own motion around the Sun and the Sun's motion along the horizon, and can be plotted over the year (Fig. 6-3). The length of time it becomes visible is short, varying from one to three weeks, and it moves in steep angles and with rapidity. A sequence of

MERCURY'S ASTRONOMICAL PROPERTIES

the appearances of Mercury over the course of the Earth year reveals six periods of visibility every two months and alternating between the eastern and western horizon (Fig. 6-4). There are actually seven appearances over the year, but the seventh is not visible. When these short sequences are combined, a helix of spiralling curves is produced (Fig. 6-5). In effect the path of Mercury around the Sun, from the perspective of Earth, describes a caduceus (see p.83).

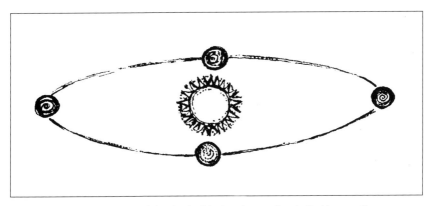

[Fig. 6.1] *Oscillation of Mercury to the left and right of the Sun when seen from the Earth's perspective.*

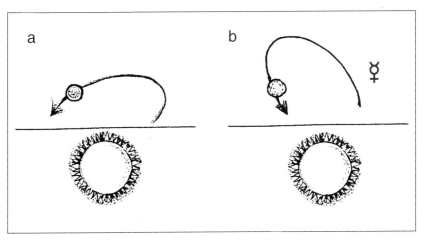

[Fig. 6.2] *Visibility of Mercury above the eastern (a) and western horizon (b).*

43

HOMOEOPATHY OF THE SOLAR SYSTEM: MERCURY

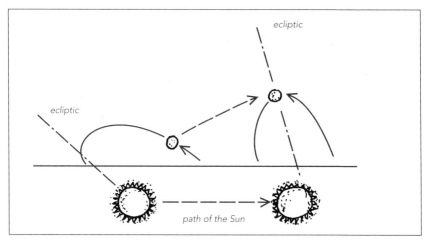

[Fig. 6.3] *Visible path of Mercury when combined with the movement of the Sun along the horizon.*

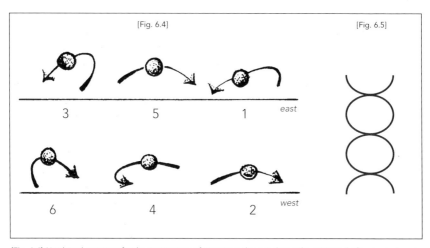

[Fig. 6.4] *Numbered sequence for the appearances of Mercury in the east during the morning (before sunrise), and the west during the evening (after sunset).* [Fig. 6.5] *Spiralling curves of Mercury's combined path as a caduceus.*

Mercury's orbit is a classic example of an ellipse, i.e. having a long and short axis. All known planets within the solar system exhibit such elliptical orbits, but Mercury being more extreme than most. Furthermore it is eccentric in that the Sun occupies one pivotal focus of this ellipse while the other focus appears empty. The orbital position when it is closest to the Sun is known as the perihelion point. The position furthest away from the Sun, at the opposite side to perihelion on the long axis of the elliptic orbit, is known as the aphelion point. The intensity of solar radiation therefore varies considerably, being 2.3 times greater at perihelion as compared to aphelion (compare this with the rapid changes of temperature in the metal remedy p.6). The polar regions appear to have areas of permanent sunlight (especially the vertical surfaces of mountains) as well as permanent shadow (at the crater bases). The temperature at these two sites would be approximately 270° C and well below 0° C respectively. Radar studies suggest there may even be collections of ice at the poles. Note that the planet has negligible axis tilt for rotation (being no more than 2°), thus variations in the angularity of the sunlight cannot occur at the poles. At the exact position of the pole, an observer with a flat horizon would see the horizon bisect the sun.

There is an approximate 4:1 ratio between the Earth's orbital period (365.25 days) and that of Mercury (eighty eight days). This is reflected in the relationship between the heart rate and the respiratory rate. Thus in normal health there should be four heartbeats to every one breath cycle (in and out breath). This ratio is due to the numerological laws pertaining to each planet. Thus four is the number for planet Earth.

Conjunctions during orbit
An upper or superior conjunction is when Mercury is on the opposite side of the Sun to the Earth (Fig. 6-6). Following this Mercury moves seemingly away from the Sun in an eastward direction. It reaches the point of greatest distance from the Sun (greatest eastern elongation) in about thirty six days. It thus becomes visible at dusk during this time, being relatively further from the Sun's glare. It then appears to approach the Sun again as it moves into inferior conjunction (moving between the Sun and the Moon). It takes twenty two days to reach this inferior conjunction and will become obscured by the Sun's light during this travel. After inferior conjunction, it continues its orbit to reach greatest western elongation in another twenty two days. During this movement

away from the Sun it becomes visible during early dawn. After this is takes thirty six days to reach superior conjunction, becoming obscured again and continuing the cycle as before. This orbit of Mercury around the Sun when considered relative to the Earth is called the synodical cycle of Mercury and lasts approximately one hundred and sixteen days.

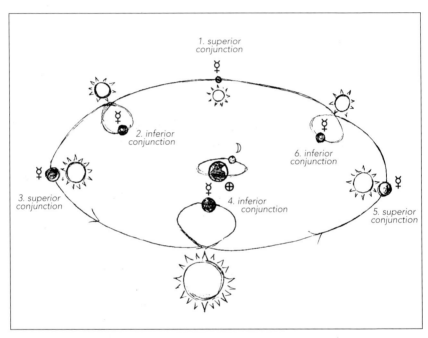

[Fig. 6.6] Mercury's synodical orbit around the Sun during one Earth year. Positions 2, 4, 6 are inferior conjunctions where Mercury lies directly between the Sun and Earth. Positions 1, 3, 5 are superior conjunctions where Mercury lies directly opposite the Sun relative to the Earth. Position 1 can enter the following year to cause four superior conjunctions in particular Earth years.

Of all the other visible planets the energy of Mercury is the most related to the Sun, due to its close proximity to the Sun. In one Earth year, Mercury completes three synodical cycles (i.e. 3 times 116 = 348 days). There are six (occasionally seven) conjunctions with the Sun, three being inferior and three superior. A hexagonal shape can be constructed from this pattern of conjunctions.

This is of relevance to the plant kingdom, where Mercury governs the leaves attached to the main stem of the plant. The stem is governed by the Sun, and the stem leaves that radiate from the stem in a whorl-like pattern are usually arranged in the same pattern as Mercury orbiting the Sun. The leaves are the organs for the breathing process in plants, which is physiologically (as in the animal and human kingdoms) a Mercury process.

Rotational speed and relationship with the orbital speed
Mercury spins around its rotational axis once in every 58.65 days. Its speed of rotation is constant throughout its orbit at 6.27° per day (equivalent Earth day). This was only discovered after radar measurements; previously it was widely believed that the period of planetary rotation was exactly equal to the orbital period. This erroneous assumption had caused the incorrect belief that Mercury always presented the same face to the Sun, the opposite side being in perpetual darkness. However the measured rotational period is exactly two-thirds of its period of orbit (Fig. 6-7). Thus there is a 2:3 ratio between its orbit and rotational spin; or in other words the planet

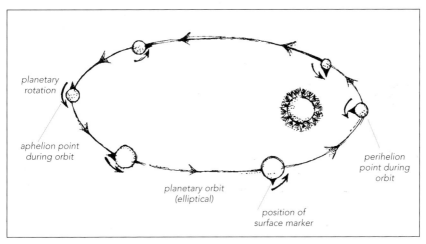

[Fig. 6.7] *Mercury's rotation:orbit ratio of 3:2 around the sun. Mercury completes a rotation on average two-thirds along each orbit around the Sun. Thus there are three planetary rotations for every two solar orbits.*

rotates on its axis three times whilst it orbits the Sun twice over. Consequently, upon successive transitions through perihelion, Mercury presents opposite faces to the Sun.

Sun retrograde, double sunset and double sunrise

The Sun exhibits a peculiar movement as witnessed from certain surface locations on Mercury and at certain points of its orbit. This can be understood after a more detailed analysis of the apparent rate of motion of the Sun as seen from Mercury. Generally planets exhibiting elliptic orbits will have a varying orbital speed according to the distance they are from the Sun. This rule is one of Kepler's Laws of Planetary Motion, which states that the area swept by the radius vector (or line) from the Sun to the planet is the same per unit time. The planet will be faster during perihelion due to the increased gravitational flux from the Sun, causing it to accelerate.

The average speed of motion of Mercury along its orbit as seen from the Sun is 4.18° per day (standard Earth day as the unit). Conversely this is the speed, as witnessed from Mercury, at which the Sun travels along the background of the zodiac belt of constellations and is the proper or true measurement of the rate of motion. It is an average value – during aphelion Mercury travels much slower at 2.81° per day and at perihelion it accelerates to 6.50° per day (as seen from the Sun).

The apparent rate of motion depends however on adjusting for the rate of rotation of Mercury – as this affects the view of the Sun from the perspective of the planet (without considering the background of zodiacal constellations for the present). Thus the average speed of the Sun as seen from Mercury becomes the difference between the latter's rate of rotation and rate of orbit, i.e. 6.27° minus 4.18°, which equals 2.09° per day. As highlighted above, this varies according to the distance Mercury is from the Sun. At aphelion (furthest away position) the Sun appears to travel at 6.27° minus 2.81°, equalling 3.46° per day. At perihelion (closest position) the Sun appears to travel at 6.27° minus 6.50°, which equals -0.23° per day.

MERCURY'S ASTRONOMICAL PROPERTIES

This negative value (albeit small) means that during perihelion passage the Sun actually stops its normal westward progress (sunrise in the east and sunset in the west) to temporarily reverse its direction of travel in the mercurian sky. It thus moves eastward slightly, then returning to its usual

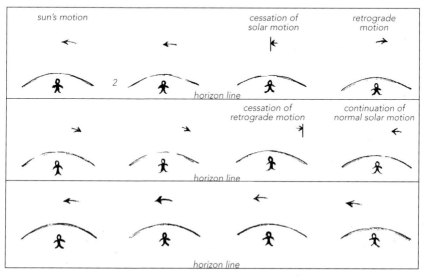

[Fig. 6.8] *Movement of the Sun as seen on Mercury at perihelion and sub-solar maximal point. The picture frames along the time-line show the Sun's motion along the Mercurian sky. The observer is facing south.*

course to set in the western horizon. This is known as a Sun retrograde and will be best observed at the point on the planet's equator directly facing the Sun (known as the perihelion subsolar point, Fig. 6-8).

Even more intriguing is the effect of this if witnessed from locations 90° east or west of the subsolar point during perihelion passage. If the observer stands at a location on the equator 90° east, during the afternoon, the Sun is seen travelling across the sky at a progressively decreasing rate and yet appearing larger and brighter as it approaches the western horizon. Just before perihelion the Sun sets, but at perihelion Mercury's increased orbital speed over its rotational speed creates the Sun retrograde effect. This leads to the Sun briefly rising above the horizon again and then setting for the second time almost immediately after (Fig. 6-9). There is a double sunset at this position 90° east! If standing at a location 90° west of the perihelion subsolar point the observer would see a very bright Sun rise slowly at dawn above the

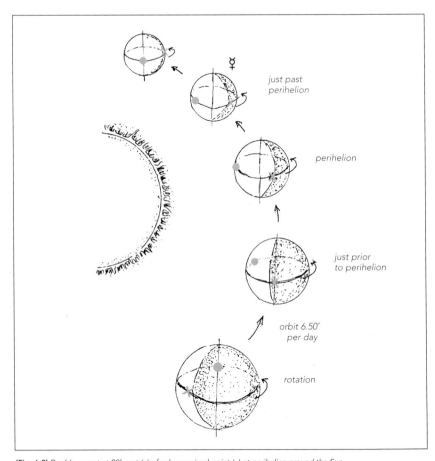

[Fig. 6.9] *Double sunset at 90° east (x) of solar maximal point (•) at perihelion around the Sun.*

eastern horizon and then stop moving, reversing to set below the horizon and then rising again (Fig. 6-10). This is a double sunrise at 90° west! It will then travel progressively faster across the sky, yet becoming smaller and fainter towards noon.

MERCURY'S ASTRONOMICAL PROPERTIES

The 3:2 ratio of rotation to orbit is also relevant to Mercury's influence on the lungs. There are three lobes forming the right lung, and two lobes forming the left lung (the heart is slightly nearer the left side of the body and takes up some of the space in the central-left side of the

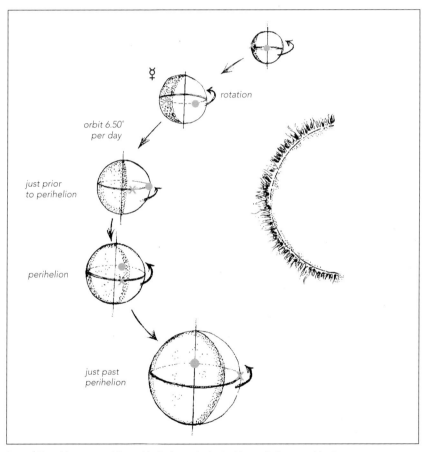

[Fig. 6.10] *Double sunrise at 90° west (×) of solar maximal point (•) at perihelion around the Sun.*

chest cavity). This difference in number of lobes allows the left and right lungs to anchor differing qualities of soul force in the breathing process. The ego consciousness is the character imbued with soul-spirit forces (to a greater or lesser degree) and incarnates more strongly though the right side of the body. The astral body (as the higher form of the emotional body) incarnates more strongly through the left side.

Relationship with the Moon orbit

Pertinent also is the close relationship between Mercury and the Moon. The Moon nearly completes four synodical cycles (4 times 29.5 days = 118 days) during one synodical cycle of Mercury, i.e. the Moon orbits around the Earth four times in the time taken for Mercury to orbit around the Sun, from the perspective of the Earth (Fig. 6-11). When considering the time difference between the synodical and sidereal revolutions of Mercury another close relationship with the Moon is revealed: 116 minus 88 gives 28 days, which is close to the sidereal revolution of the Moon (27.36 days, or the time taken by the Moon to span the zodiac once over and return to its starting point). In terms of consciousness, the sidereal cycle of Mercury represents the communication between Mercury and the rest of the cosmos, enabling Mercury to convey messages between the wider cosmos and our solar system. The synodical cycle represents the relationship Mercury has with the Earth in relaying the blueprints from the Sun into the Earth material realm. By completing one sidereal orbit between these two cycles of Mercury the Moon can be seen to mediate the cosmic function of Mercury with its earthly duties. The Moon enables the cosmic Mercury to relate to the Earth realm, especially with regard to the unconscious and subconscious realms of Earth. In other words Mercury requires the Moon in order to mediate its messages into the unconscious and subconscious realms of Earth and the human population.

Temperature fluctuations due to orbit and rotation

When Mercury is closest to the Sun, it is extremely hot, at 740° K (467° C) for the regions facing the Sun most directly. However the night side facing away from the Sun may not actually be lit for months at a time, due to Mercury's slow rotation. This side can actually be one of the coolest places in the solar system at 90° K (−183° C). (Note how sensitive the patient is to both heat and cold in the homoeopathic materia medica picture.)

MERCURY'S ASTRONOMICAL PROPERTIES

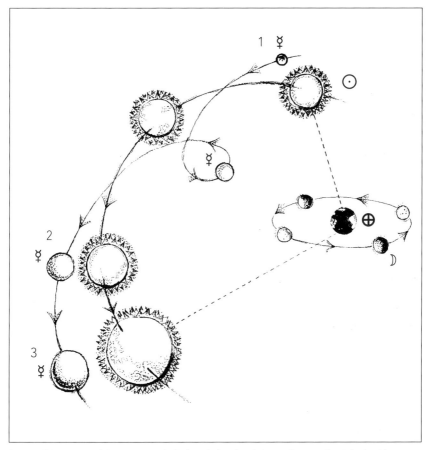

[Fig. 6.11] *Comparison of the Moon's synodical orbit with the orbit of Mercury. During eighty-eight days (almost one-quarter of an Earth year) Mercury completes one orbit of the Sun (1 → 2) in its sidereal cycle. Thus it returns to the same position relative to the Sun. The Moon's synodical orbit around the Earth is shown (2 → 3) with the movement of Mercury also during this time (2 → 3). Mercury's movement from 1 → 3 is its synodical orbit.*

Evolution of the rotational speed

Mercury had a much faster rotational spin in its ancient past. Scientists do not yet know how or why it slowed down to its present slow rotational period, but theorised it did so within five hundred million years of its initial formation. It slowed down when evolution on Earth was required to slow down. Compared to the spiritual realm, the pace of life on Earth in the third-dimension is very slow. Linear time enables events to be slowed down and thus magnified, allowing human souls to focus for long periods on the same project or lesson. The blueprints relayed down to Earth though the portal of Mercury had also to therefore be slowed down to limit the frequency of evolutionary and transformative triggers from outer space. As the Earth ascends, linear time is speeding and collapsing, (as shown by the increased pace of life). Mercury will follow suit by also shifting its orbital behaviour – not necessarily by speeding up. There are presently occult or hidden planets between the Sun and Mercury that may instead become exposed (including Vulcan, which is portrayed in 'Homoeopathy of the Solar System: Vulcan' within this series). Also, metallic Mercury will eventually come to solidify on planet Earth, altering its properties markedly.

Surface appearance

The surface of Mercury has been partially visually mapped by Mariner 10 during its flights past the planet in 1974-5 and appears very similar to that of the Moon, with many craters. There are broadly two types of terrain, the highlands and the lowland plains. The highlands have multiple craters with some smooth plains between heavily cratered regions. Overall there are far fewer craters on Mercury than on the Moon.

The smooth areas between craters also indicate some re-surfacing event occurred after the early bombardment that is presumed to have caused the cratering. These smooth plains have obliterated the smaller craters that would be expected to occur between the larger ones. The smooth intercrater plains are very similar in reflective light analysis to the lowland smooth plains in other parts of the planet, suggesting common events leading to both. Theories include molten rock from internal volcanic eruption, or molten rock from the impact of external bodies.

Of significance here is Mercury fulminate, a form used in the manufacture of explosives and which can explode upon impact. This energy is related to the crater formation on Mercury, and is due to the disparity between blueprints coming out of the spiritual realm when they impact on too dense a material realm. Mercury would normally seek to guide new information into the planet gracefully and provide for relatively easy transformation. However the nature of evolution on the material realm encouraged sudden and cataclysmic transformations. For example, the known evolution of physical forms in the animal kingdom of Earth has been studded with sudden departure and inception of species, as well as sudden and destructive events such as plague, massive flooding, ice formation and so on. Similarly Mercury often ensures there is a jarring of the new blueprints upon entering the material realm, with potentially explosive consequences for the inhabitants of the planet.

Molten rock from volcanoes and external impact bodies are both potentially involved in formation of the smooth plains. If the crater was to be compared to a syphilitic ulcer (which is a distortion of a physiological Mercury process), it is common to find debris adherent to the surface of the ulcer (see p.153). This slough is a collection of firm pus and exudate, containing dead white blood cells, syphilitic bacteria, fluid secretions and connective scar tissue. It represents the decay of the old obsolete blueprint information held by the white cells. The syphilitic bacterium looks remarkably similar to a spiralling caduceus and to the waves of metatronic energy. This is the spiralling of subtle forces from the spiritual realm to the material realm and vice versa. Along the pranic tube representing the subtle forces of the spinal cord there are analogous sinusoidal currents of electrical, magnetic and gravitational energies, also depicted as Ida, Pingali and the Sushumna currents in Yogic knowledge. The spirochete or spiral syphilitic bacteria (called Treponema pallidum, see p.153) represents stuck spiritual information not able to enter and penetrate the material tissues of that body. The slough that is in the way represents an immunological block created within the human organism to prevent proper cellular communion with the spiritual realm. The microcosm of human physiology and pathology reflects the macrocosm of the world and the cosmos. Hence the smooth slough covering the craters and the lowland plains of Mercury are formed by the combination of turbulent comet impact energy with dense volcanic melt activity within the planet. This is the spiritual message (by way of comet impact) having a turbulent effect on the stuck old and obsolete blueprints within the planet's interior.

The craters represent the energy of cavitation and tubulation as regards the flow of astral and higher spiritual energy. When spiritual energy penetrates the material plane, there is a penetrating current which causes tubes, craters and hollow chambers to form within the material substance. Mercury is the classic planet to receive these currents by way of blueprints and passes these onto the Earth material plane. The Moon works in association with Mercury to feed these blueprints into the subconsciousness of the Earth planetary system. However, when the fall of humanity occurred, leading to a separation of the consciousness of humanity from the divine world, many axiotonal lines of light and spiritual current were cut off from human bodies and souls. This led to the human soul and body having various programs of ageing, degeneration and physical limitation. The covering of the craters of Mercury as an event represents this sealing over of the divine connection. It also reflects the workings of the syphilitic miasm, whereby events become hidden, sealed over and ulcers (c.f. craters) become internalised.

The largest crater event is at the Caloris basin of the planet, which spans 1340 km and comprises ulceration of the surface with a mountainous terrain of huge rocks. This region is near one of the hot spots on the planet (where the most intense solar radiation occurs at perihelion); hence its name. It is considered to be due to the impact of an enormous object probably about 3.85 billion years ago. Due to the shock waves travelling through the planet from this event there is an irregular area of jumbled rocks at the antipode or exact opposite point of the planet where the ground was shaken violently from the focus of the merged seismic shock waves. The creation of this crater occurred at a significant time in the history of Earth. Prior to this, the Earth had a softer gel-like structure. There were also three main kingdoms of nature – the human/animal, animal/plant and plant/mineral kingdoms, with composite hybrid species (see 'Homoeopathy of the Solar System: Moon and Silver' in this series). The energy and substance of the Moon was largely bound with that of Earth, only later did it separate to form a satellite in orbit around Earth. After the Caloris event, the Earth began to harden and to properly develop as a dense mineralised body. Metals, minerals and rocks solidified from liquid states and the nature kingdoms segregated into the four kingdoms of human, animal, plant and mineral that exist presently.

Another mercurian feature found in the Mariner 10 pictures that science presently has difficulty explaining is the abundant and intricate network of lobate scarps throughout the surface. These are deep slopes and ridges in the landscape arranged in lobular and geometrical patterns. They are thought to be compression faults due to some shrinkage episode of the planet – which may have caused as much as a 4 km of reduction of its diameter. The reason for this shrinkage is hypothesised to be due to cooling of the planet or a change in its rotation. It is interesting however to compare the presence of tall mountainous ranges and heaped up boulders interspersed with deep crater bases and surface faults with the role Mercury plays in mythology. He transverses the Olympian and heavenly realms high above mountain-tops as well as the deeply subterranean chambers of the underworld (see p.87). It is as if the very landscape of Mercury mirrors the dichotomy and polarisation of the superconscious and subconscious realms of humankind. The shrinkage of Mercury correlated with the densification and mineralisation of Earth during late Lemuria – for at this time the consciousness of humanity also became segregated into layers of subconsciousness, waking consciousness and superconscious. This required Mercury to guide the human souls along the pathways of travel for consciousness between their incarnations and during sleep – resonating with compression and a change in the very structure of Mercury the planet.

Iron core and magnetic field

Mercury has a mass calculated at 3.3 x 10^{26} grams and a mean density of 5.43g/cm^3. This is very similar to the bulk densities of Earth (5.5) and Venus (5.2) but much greater than that of Mars (3.9). It is thought that

Mercury contains about 70% iron to provide for such a mass and density, the rest being silica-based material. Mercury also has its own magnetic field which science currently cannot explain. The planet has too slow a rotation to create such a field. Conceivably molten iron circulating within the interior of the planet could provide a dynamo effect and thus explain the magnetic field. But it is thought that the long period for cooling of the planet has by now solidified most if not all the interior iron. This magnetic field also protects the planet from the intense solar wind of ionised particles bombarding its surface.

However spiritual principles are required to understand energetic fields, including magnetism. Energy cannot be explained by simply transposing material events and the interactions of material substances with each other. Rather the converse, that material substances and processes can only be explained by understanding the subtle energetic interactions between them. Energy can exist outside and outwith matter. Thus the magnetic field of Mercury is a consequence of its interaction with other planets, the Sun and the wider cosmos of stars. Its field can interact with the magnetic fields of distant stars, and such interaction is one basis for communication of blueprints between the two.

The laws of magnetism are as yet very poorly understand by humanity, and myriad angels and spiritual beings are involved in regulating the subtle but powerful magnetic fields of stellar bodies. Magnetism especially conveys forces of will-power and the first ray, which is closely aligned to the Father and Will aspect of God as Trinity. Mercury's iron substance provides a firm anchoring of these subtle forces into our solar system. Iron is the metal for incarnation of will forces, and provides the metal substrate for inception of such energies deep into the physical realm and physical body. Iron also enables a breathing process, for it easily binds to cosmic energy and guides this into the planetary core, where the cosmic energy is released. The iron then circulates back to the surface providing fresh substrate for further cosmic energy. Similarly the human lungs cannot function without iron in the red blood cells. Mercury rules the breathing process and the environment of the lungs. As Mercury guides inward the prana or energy contained within the inspired air, this fresh energy must be received by the capillary blood sent from the right side of the heart.

The iron of Mercury is vibrationally resonating with the iron of the planets Earth and Venus. Martian iron has a very different focus to the iron of these other three planets. Whereas Martian iron is focused on reaching toward far-flung cosmic stations, the iron of Earth is a focus for reception and incarnation. Mercury is responsible for channelling this cosmic impulse sent from Mars toward and into the Earth. The iron within Mercury is intimately affected by the iron of Earth; the fact there is no material connection between the two deposits of iron is not of relevance – for an energy travels between the two. This energy carries the blueprint information Mercury is transmitting to Earth. (Further details can be found in 'Homoeopathy of the Solar System: Mars and Iron' in this series.)

The atmosphere

Until recently Mercury was considered to be without an atmosphere. Nonetheless one that has been discovered is largely composed of oxygen, sodium and potassium, with some hydrogen and helium. Science considers the first three constituents perhaps arising from vaporised rock when small comets hit the planet's surface. It is interesting to note that the sodium:potassiumn ratio in the mercurian air is 60:1, compared to a 4:1 ratio on the Earth Moon. Hydrogen and helium are thought to arise from charged particles within the solar wind becoming captured within the magnetic field of the planet and changing into neutral atoms. Some atoms have sufficient velocity to escape the planet, but enough remain to create a thin atmosphere.

However, an atmosphere is formed essentially before the solid phase as a planet densifies out of the etheric realm. The material realm is only the last densified manifestation of energy already in existence in the spiritual realm. Of note sodium and potassium ions in the atmosphere would scatter solar photons very efficiently and radio-based telescopes easily see these energetic emissions.

HOMOEOPATHY OF THE SOLAR SYSTEM: MERCURY

Even more so, however, the atmospheric sodium and potassium provide a material basis for the astral plane on Mercury. The astral plane is the fourth-dimensional plane above the third-dimension of material manifestation. It is analogous to the plane of reality where souls travel using their astral bodies during sleep/dreaming. It is also the plane through which souls transit when leaving the physical realm to return to the spiritual between incarnations, i.e. after death of the physical vehicle. However many souls who have left their dead physical bodies become stuck by karmic memories within the lower astral plane. This lower level contains the emotional debris of humanity and appears like energetic smog which clouds the proper communication of signals between the third-dimensional Earth surface and the cosmic spiritual realms above it. Various discarnate entities reside here, such as demons, vampires, etheric shells of former physical bodies (ghosts) and stuck human soul fragments. On the other hand, the higher levels of the astral plane contain angel academies, libraries of Akashic records, spirit guides, nature spirits and so on. The astral plane can be felt as a constantly shifting realm of energy and emotional flow. Emotions, sensations and desires are visibly manifest as charged streams of energy, which cause attraction or repulsion between objects and beings within the astral plane. Events can move very quickly or slowly in this plane and thus time and space becomes distorted. This flow consciousness provides for the dream experiences of humans whereby many lifetimes of dream-like experiences can occur in the space of a few minutes.

The planet Mercury is responsible for providing a clear channel for information to transit the astral plane of Earth and reach the surface inhabitants. Many times in Earth's past, as well as obviously prevalent at present, there occurs distortion of these spiritual and cosmic signals. This distortion is due to the smog-like effect of humanity's emotional debris within the lower astral plane, causing deviation of the signals as they transit. In Mercury, the astral plane has not been segregated from the third-dimension as it has on Earth. If one were standing on Mercury the astral plane would be directly perceivable with the physical senses. Events and happenings within the astral plane are clear picture images in the atmosphere of the planet. The very atmosphere holds the astral plane in material and physical form. Sodium is one of the mineral carriers for astral energy in a planet. Thus its rich presence in the blood is a sign of the strong astral impulses working through this fluid, imbuing it with life force. Potassium on the other hand is a carrier for etheric vitality forces, as evident by its rich content in plant material. The much greater amount of sodium in the mercurian atmosphere is a sign of the strong anchoring of astral vibration within the air. This can be compared to the relative preponderance of potassium on the Moon, which has a much more vegetative and nurturing relationship with the Earth. This is evident also by potassium being rich in plant tissue and conducting a similarly unconscious role within the human body metabolism compared to the much more dynamic and awake quality of sodium processes.

In the future this atmospheric astral physical picture consciousness will also become prevalent on Earth. Humans are not yet ready to withstand the shifts of consciousness needed to be able to physically see the realities of the astral plane whilst also in their physical bodies in the third-dimension. This would equate to the situation of a lucid dream but even more so, when a soul wakes up to an almost fully alert consciousness whilst in the dream state. This situation is gradually changing on Earth through the collapse of the boundaries between the dimensions. Earth is merging the third- and fourth-dimensions, and fairly rapidly entering deeper levels of the fifth-dimension. This is evident by the faster flow of life events, greater emotional expression of humans and the increased communication and information technology on the planet.

Chapter 7

Mercury and the Cabalah of number

The Cabalah is said to have developed within the Jewish faith in the regions of Egypt and Palestine during the birth of Christianity. The book of the Cabalah contains detailed instructions and techniques guiding the soul on its return path to spirit. It describes an alphabet of symbols through letters and numbers. The language created enables communication between beings in different dimensions – between humans and the spiritual realm. Through it the disciple can make direct contact with spirit guides, angels, gods and other entities.

Gematria

There are several techniques of interpretation within the Cabalah, used to find the hidden or esoteric meaning of any given word. Gematria is a method used to find the numerical value of a word. Words having the same value can have an important spiritual relationship and be explanatory of each other. For the English language a number (called the alpha number) is given for each letter of the alphabet:

Letter	Alpha number	Letter	Alpha number	Letter	Alpha number	Letter	Alpha number
A	1	H	8	O	15	V	22
B	2	I	9	P	16	W	23
C	3	J	10	Q	17	X	24
D	4	K	11	R	18	Y	25
E	5	L	12	S	19	Z	26
F	6	M	13	T	20		
G	7	N	14	U	21		

[Fig. 7.1] *Table of Gematria alpha numbers for the English alphabet*

The numbers for each letter of the word being analysed undergo addition, but not completely to a single digit as in other systems of numerology. There are several means of arranging the numbers thus derived, e.g.

GOD = G + O + D = 7 + 15 + 4 = 7154 as well as 26 in gematria.

With reference to Hermes as a name for Mercury, the calculation is:

HERMES = 8 + 5 + 18 + 13 + 5 + 19 = 68

Words that have the same value under gematria include the following:

LOGOS
GOD SELF
A SOUL
PILLAR
GILGUL

Below are some of the essential characteristics of Hermes/Mercury through the related words.

Logos
Logos (pl. logi) is the term describing the consciousness ensouling a great structure such as a planet, a star, a galaxy or a universe. This being functions in an administrative capacity, holding the energy field of a system in place across dimensions of reality throughout linear time so as to integrate the myriad experiences within that system. The logos is rather like a scaffold or framework providing a stable movement of energy within the structure. This spiritual being has characteristics peculiar to itself and follows its own destiny, yet is bound to the destiny of souls living within the structure. Individual souls incarnating within a planet, for instance, are living and moving within such a being. This should not be confused with the energy field and consciousness of the body of the planet itself, for example Earth consciousness is often called Earth Mother and Gaia (being a female planet). Until recent changes in the spiritual hierarchy and

spiritual administration of Earth amongst the Ascended Masters, the logos ensouling Earth was Sanat Kumara. He had received a long period of training (over billions of years) on planet Venus, in preparation for his role on Earth. Sanat Kumara is now moving to another level of activity within the galaxy and the job of Earth planetary logos is presently partly undertaken by the Buddha. Mercury has the key role of guiding messages from the level of the spiritual hierarchy and the logos to incarnated souls on the third-dimension surface of Earth. Eventually the human soul realises its true spiritual nature and is able to activate the logoic level of collective spiritual consciousness within (see Fig. 7-2). This is a particularly elevated lightbody (or spiritual body) which enables the disciple to make planet or global level decisions for collective humanity. The greater responsibility this entails can only be satisfied through unconditional love for humanity and a willingness to be of service to the process of Earth ascension.

God self
The path to enlightenment is not one for the faint of heart. It involves courage to become truly co-creative and activate the God spark within, the God self. At the essential and highest level of one's spirit there is union with God. At-one-ment leads to the state of an infinite soul. It is also a Mahatma consciousness, whereby the soul is at one with All That Is and is all present and all knowing. During this long journey the soul must accept and develop its individuality. There can be no dependency on spirit guides and angels even for life-affirming decisions. The disciple must learn to take higher level decisions that impact on collective consciousness and the divine plan. It takes on more and more spiritual responsibility. Mercury the psychopomp and guiding god no longer becomes an external messenger from the spiritual realm. He becomes the Mercury within and (as Hermes in this Cabalistic formula) activates the ability to receive spiritual messages directly into the subtle and physical bodies. The disciple has become a direct channel to the spiritual realm (Fig. 7-3).

MERCURY AND THE CABALAH OF NUMBER

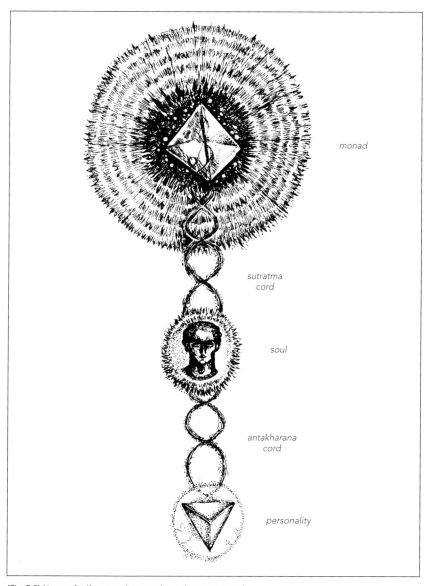

[**Fig. 7.2**] *Nature of self as monad, personality and intervening soul.*
The Monad forms the upper triad of astral, mental and spiritual energy. The personality forms the lower triad of physical, emotional and lower mental energy. The soul integrates the two triads with cords of energy. The sutratma cord links soul to monad. The antakharana links soul to personality. Eventually the monad, soul and personality merge as one and the two cords become fused.

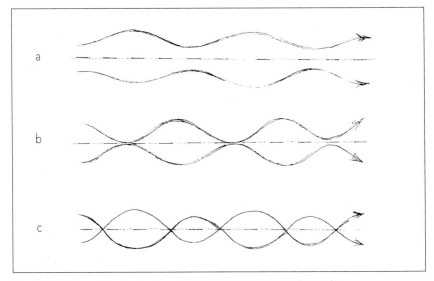

[Fig. 7.3] *Spiralling energies of varying stages of integration between monad and personality.*
(a) is the undeveloped brute where no integration occurs between monadic energy and the incarnated personalities.
(b) reveals interfacing between the two streams of consciousness and is the usual state for the average human.
(c) shows greater and deepening integration between monad and personalities for the disciple on the spiritual path to self-realisation.

A soul
This term portrays the uniqueness of each soul. Although each soul has infinite possibilities of action and experience, not all souls are equal in what they have chosen to achieve. The soul learns to break from dependency with other souls within the pool of humanity. During the early rounds of Earth evolution souls had a sense of harmony and one-ness with the rest of human race. During incarnations such souls would experience strong familial, tribal and community ties. Indeed an angel would be recruited from the spiritual realm to oversee each grouping of humanity. Family angels, tribal angels and community angels became so deeply entrenched that individuality became very difficult to develop within the personality – out of fear of breaking from traditional values. These traditions served a useful purpose – to develop soul groupings and karmic experiences between souls. However the karmic ties now

require rescission (a return to the state of alignment with the spiritual realm). This liberates each soul from the debris of shared karma within the collective. Mercury reveals his ability to honour and provide integrity to the soul as an individual having a unique personal biography. Mercury is cognisant of each soul's personal karma, relationships and destiny.

Pillar
The pillar is a strong vertical support. It symbolises the strength and integrity of the spinal cord and vertebral bony column, supporting the physical body into a vertical alignment. The uprightness of character is directly related to the strength of the spine and the pranic tube underlying the physical structure (see p.208). Through Mercury, spine and pranic tubal defects can be rectified. However two pillars also represent a doorway into alternate realities, a multi-dimensional gateway represented by the zodiac sign Gemini (see p.76). Mercury is the god of travelling and the spiritual journey is many times beset by decisions with very little conscious guidance. Mercury generally works behind the scenes to instil a sense of the right path to the traveller, without fostering awareness of the source of this information nor dependency on the guidance. Spirit often creates situations where there are several possibilities of action, creating confusion in the soul so as to develop courage and a sense of discovery along the path.

Gilgul
This is the Hebrew word for 'reincarnation'. As the psychopomp, Mercury has a direct influence on the stages between earthly incarnations of the soul. After the death of the physical body the soul enters a bardo state between lives where it rapidly re-experiences its biography thus far (see p.92). Without Mercury the soul is unable to properly review its former lives nor develop its plans for the following incarnations.

Chapter 8

Mercury in astrology and psychology

Basic themes

Those influenced by Mercury have a quick sharp mind. They rapidly grasp ideas behind situations and projects and act promptly on their insights. They appear to move with grace and speed through projects. However they can be very difficult to pin down and often appear elusive. The child is a quick developer, learning to talk, walk and take an interest in things at an early age. They have a genuine interest in many things.

However they can become deceptive, lie and make up stories to their own advantage. They may steal from others and become very attracted to other people's property, even becoming kleptomaniac (with a compulsive need to covet other's possessions). They can become con-artists, tricksters and sociopaths – and usually use cleverness and the gift of the gab to manipulate situations rather than brute force or aggression.

They can be unconventional, taking a unique route through things and preferring to find their own methods rather than copy others. They can be opportunistic, taking advantage of situations and seizing gains the moment they arise.

In relationships they can appear callous and heartless, going from one partner to another and making excuses to hide their unfaithfulness. Commitment can be difficult for them.

They can appear as gifted guides and counsellors and become a seeker of truth in spiritual matters. They are fascinated by the mysteries of death and the afterlife, as well as magic and alchemy. They are usually not content to follow one path, but find the truth behind many in an integrative fashion.

Mercury retrograde

Retrograde occurs three or four times a year when, from a geocentric (Earth-centred) perspective, the Sun is apparently moving faster than Mercury for a short period. Therefore Mercury appears to be travelling slower than its average speed during this period. Alternatively Mercury appears to move more slowly relative to the Earth. In terms of an astrological reading, the retrograde process does not start and stop at the actual stationary points, but before and after them respectively. The stationary points are where the speed of Mercury is roughly equal to that of Earth, thus the motion of Mercury appears momentarily 'frozen'. At these times a special energy arises, but the effects of retrograde appear beforehand and continue afterwards for a phase when the average speed between the two planets is still in the process of change. Thus there are several phases within the retrograde period:

- The first phase is the end of the previous Mercury cycle; it has slowed down and then travelled through a stationary point as it starts to enter the stage of inferior conjunction.

- The second phase is during and soon after inferior conjunction, lasting until Mercury starts speeding again.

- The third phase when Mercury reaches the second stationary point (also called stationary direct) and is leaving the stage of inferior conjunction, entering extreme lateral declination again and starting to enter the stage of superior conjunction.

There are myriad happenings on Earth associated with the retrograde energy of Mercury, and these include:

- Misplaced or lost messages and communications, in whatever format, e.g. letters, emails, telephone messages and so on.

- A misunderstanding between people at all levels of social interaction.

- People feel a general pessimism, defeatism, apathy and negative thinking.

- Computer 'crashes' and malfunctions. Viral attacks on computers.

- Electrical or other failures of machines, e.g. telephone answering machines, camcorders, video-players, cars and so on.

- Meetings becoming cancelled, rescheduled unexpectedly, forgotten or delayed.

- Tasks or projects started just before or during a retrograde period create more trouble than they are worth. Energies become scattered, people get distracted and nothing gets done.

- Planning out things becomes confusing, thus people often cannot define their aims; they put 'the cart before the horse' and cannot 'see the wood for the trees'.

- Missing or failing important deadlines in tasks and projects.

- Delayed childbirth.

- Confusion in mental processes, poor examination or mental performance.

There is a widespread belief that the effects of Mercury retrograde are generally malefic and that it is best to be patient and still. It is generally agreed amongst astrologers that no new or major task should be undertaken during this period. However in this position Mercury reveals dysfunction in energy. The cause of difficulty is not in Mercury, but rather in the experience of the soul from prior action and expectation. If there was an inherent defect in the machine, or an underlying communication problem between people, it would be revealed, but not caused by, a Mercury retrograde position.

During Mercury's usual course in space, it conveys the perception of time in a linear fashion – thus events are perceived as arising from past to present and thence to the future. During the retrograde phase linear time (and space) is unplugged, and a gateway is opened in the soul's consciousness to perceiving the true non-linearity of time. Events from the past and the future can flood into the present moment and be felt as all happening at once. Signals therefore become entangled, but the retrograde period shows the soul novel or unusual perspectives for constructively dealing with the situation at hand. If the soul is working through a poorly developed personality then such insights are usually constrained to the past and future lives of the soul. The more developed the alignment between soul and personality the more information can enter from the unconscious and subconscious of collective humanity and world memory. At even more developed levels of soul enlightenment, there is information received from cosmic memory and distant stars, through the portal of Mercury within the solar system.

Many would experience this information as an opportunity to pause, reflect and re-organise their life. If these inner impulses are not heeded then the destructive and inhibitory aspects of the retrograde may manifest to stop any erroneously chosen blind path from being followed. During a retrograde, meditation can bring deeper insights than before and the outer world may actually slow down temporarily in one's field of awareness. When Mercury returns to direct orbit around the Sun, the soul should act upon the influences received during the retrograde, bringing about materialisation.

Benefits can therefore be gleaned from a retrograde if the soul can open to the new possibilities rather than focus on any loss. These include:

- Projects and plans take on novel and interesting directions that prove profitable in some way.

- Old antiquated information or belief systems are updated. Mistakes from the past are corrected.

- Unfinished tasks and projects from the past are completed, especially those started or planned during a previous Mercury retrograde period which now become activated in the present retrograde.

- New practical energy comes into manifestation and with it newfound zeal and enthusiasm.

- Research into new fields accelerates during this time.

- Travelling is particularly rewarding during this period. New discoveries and unexpected events lead to more interesting journeys which depart from the prior plan or usual routine.

- Old karmic patterns can surface to be finally released, and after the initial difficulty, the soul feels more liberated.

The phases of retrograde motion can be summarised thus:

- During the first phase as described above, with slow entry into retrograde, the energy of the soul is blocked from projecting into the future. Unfinished, karmic or unresolved issues can flood the present consciousness from the past. Most people feel thrown off balance, unable to go forward with their plans.

- During the second phase of actual inferior conjunction, lasting approximately twenty-two days, a creative window of consciousness is opened into the past and future. Intuition is clearer.

- During the third phase, as Mercury leaves the retrograde period, the energy formerly from the past now recedes, providing a path for consciousness to project into the future. Here is an opportunity to plan ahead, to organise and implement what has been learnt. Momentum is given to the new ideas as Mercury picks up speed.

Personality types when Mercury is direct in the natal chart

Mercury direct refers to the stage of Mercury's orbit when it is travelling in superior conjunction (see p.45) and appears to be faster than the Sun from the Earth perspective. This lasts approximately thirty six days. People born with Mercury in direct phase at the time of their birth will have a different energy of Mercury working within their psyche than those born during a Mercury retrograde period. In terms of the timeline, Mercury direct conveys a firm sense of future time to the personality. Only a vague sense of coming out of the past will be generally perceived. Thus ideas and thoughts are referenced to the future, and the personality tends to project and plan ahead. They also tend to not realise where the ideas originally stemmed from in terms of the past, and have a tendency to be self-sufficient or independent in their thinking – due to a inner block to gnostic perception of ancient wisdom. Gnosticism is the thinking mode of being able to perceive ancient wisdom within present belief systems. Their ability to think directly and for the future does not necessarily mean such people are effective – for that depends on what they plan and how grounded are other elements of their soul-spiritual life.

Personality types when Mercury is retrograde in the natal chart

Imagine the mode within which consciousness works with respect to how the personality perceives the origin of its ideas. The sense of living beings from the past as the origin of their present ideas is strong when Mercury is retrograde. These beings can be aspects of the person itself, individual past lives, other human souls from their respective past lives, higher spiritual beings or guides stemming from past time co-ordinates. The present personality therefore does not feel such ideas in their mind to be their own and often has the attitude of honouring the past (such as praising their ancestors). The personality also tends to make inquiries of others rather than depend on their own inner intuition or intellect.

On the other hand, the future appears much more uncertain to this personality type than when born under Mercury direct – because the future is not easy to reference within the mental body. Also the future is dependent on the activities of the same beings from the past that the soul is conscious of, as the source of the original ideas. The soul, being in constant inner and outer dialogue with myriad beings, conducts to its personality or ego structure this sense of making decisions with reference to others. This can however lead to a difficulty in making decisions independently or with any great certainty, although it does tend to provide greater creativity and exploration of the future possibilities that can arise. The method of learning tends to be to copy others until one's own method is found. They prefer to practice. Also the personality may experience low confidence, mental confusion, poor learning abilities and difficulty planning for the future. The Mercury direct soul on the other hand avoids letting the personality realise the state of collective decision making with other beings, and provides a much more independent structure to one's character with greater innovation. However the Mercury direct personality is at risk of becoming too independent, leading to 'wrong' decision making and a haphazard future state of affairs.

Planetary rulership of the zodiacal signs

The zodiac is a belt of constellations providing the cosmic backdrop to the apparent passage of the Sun around the Earth. This is a geocentric perspective, compared to the heliocentric perspective whereby the Earth travels around the Sun. In traditional mundane astrology there are twelve zodiacal constellations, from Aries to Pisces. Each sign has a planet within the solar system that acts in rulership. In effect the ruling planet functions to interface the messages from the cosmic level (i.e. the zodiacal constellation) to the native (person concerned) of the astrological chart. Slight deviation of the rotational orbit of the Earth has led to the astrological zodiacal signs no longer matching the actual constellations present in the background. This is known as the precession of the equinox. Nonetheless astrological readings often reveal remarkably accurate insights into the character of the native.

There are three levels of rulership according to the developmental stage of the soul. If the astrological chart is analysed with respect to a lower level of rulership, then the conclusions reached may well not explain the life events of the native. Each sign within the zodiac has a mundane planetary ruler, a soul oriented (or esoteric) ruler and a hierarchical ruler. The mundane planetary ruler is that which is traditionally regarded. It defines the planet involved in the influence of the zodiac sign at the level of personality. This planet affects the relationships, external material experiences and earthly attachments of that person. The planet is invariably functioning from a viewpoint of duality with right and wrong, good and bad and the morals of society as part of its agenda.

During the spiritual path, the disciple learns to live from the level of soul, integrating this with the lower personality. Desires and attachments are overcome and the soul lives more out of service and the need for constant self-development. This is when the esoteric planetary ruler for each zodiacal sign becomes activated. The planets now work deeper into the psyche and internal dynamic of the person. Less is the soul influenced by the external world around them, but becomes sensitive to the inner spiritual world.

Eventually the soul has integrated sufficiently to merge with its spirit. This imparts greater levels of service to humanity and to the process of Earth ascension. The soul becomes a channel for more rarefied and subtle cosmic and spiritual energy. This is the stage of activation of the hierarchical planetary ruler for each zodiacal sign. The planets now function at a level of collective consciousness and the individual is accessing very pure vibrational characteristics of them.

Below is a table of the levels of rulership for Mercury.

Levels of rulership for Mercury	Zodiac sign
Mundane	Gemini and Virgo
Esoteric	Aries
Hierarchical	Scorpio

[Fig. 8.1] *Table of planetary levels of rulership for Mercury in astrology.*

Gemini
This is the zodiac sign typical of the modern information age within humanity. It governs rapid and unstable mental processes, unpredictable changes in life and relationships and a general lack of focus or cohesion. The person with Mercury ruling at the mundane position in this sign tends to learn through relating with others, through communication and educational processes with the external world. A negative portrayal of Mercury working through this sign has the closest resemblance to the mental symptoms of the materia medica picture of Mercurius.

As the disciple continues on the path, the esoteric rulership of Gemini comes to the fore as the planet Venus. This is further discussed in 'Homoeopathy of the Solar System: Venus and Copper' in this book series. Essentially Venus imparts a new level of creativity and integration between the lower self and higher self as well as integrating the sacral chakra with the throat and brow chakras. Mercury works closely with the Venusian impulse (see pp.103, 185 for the relationship between Hermes and Aphrodite).

Virgo
This is the sign where the person learns to manifest their Christ self within the external material realm. It involves dedication to service work and synthesis of aspects of self that are disharmonious with other aspects. Virgoans tend to work well within groups and communities and to cultivate the qualities of grace and devotion needed for this. They often try to find their proper place within the scheme of things, with a need to fulfil their life's purpose through work. Mercury as the mundane ruler provides this ability to work for the collective, to be enthusiastic about helping others. When the disciple activates the esoteric planetary rulers, the Moon leads the way in Virgo. This enables the surfacing of subconscious and collective patterns within the disciple. There is improved grounding of emotional energy with externalisation and manifestation of the Christ impulse into greater levels of planetary service.

Aries

Mercury is the esoteric ruler for this sign. The usual mundane ruler is Mars, who provides the zealous enthusiasm and assertiveness typical of the Arian, the person strongly expressing will and power. At this lower dualistic level of functioning there is often a need to overcome others on the material plane. At a higher subtle level of functioning the key quality becomes initiation and the ability to directly receive messages from the logoic plane of spirit (where intent and will reside). This provides the ideal framework for Mercury, imbuing Aries with messages from the spiritual and cosmic realm, especially from the higher mind and will of God. Aries can then stimulate courage and co-creativity in the disciple to receive evolutionary impulses, often never before brought into manifestation on Earth. The role of Aries is then to lead others into groundbreaking new ventures, becoming a sign for initiative and courage.

Scorpio

Mercury is the hierarchical ruler for this sign. This is its originating energy from the cosmos. Out of the constellation of Scorpio the mercurian impulse arises in its purest form. The main or alpha star in Scorpio (the visibly brightest) is Antares, which functions at a deep subconscious plane of reality. The beings of Antares were required during their evolution to understand the forces within the unconscious and subconscious planes. In doing so they developed awareness of the abdominal chakras, the nature of the hara or power centres that etherically link an incarnated being to its planet's power centres and the journey within the elemental and subterranean realms between surface incarnations. This is the overall energy radiating from Scorpio and is suitably guided into the solar system by Mercury.

As the spiritual disciple overcomes the lower personality and activates more refined aspects of the internal Mercury process the external Mercury channels greater levels of the energy from Scorpio. Invariably the disciple is functioning at a collective level on behalf of humanity. This involves the ability, indeed the requirement, to journey into the subconscious realm of humanity and into subterranean Earth. Effectively the disciple merges with the being of Mercury. There arises the power to alter these realms and re-write the history of the planet and humanity, an illustration of the magical and alchemical faculty inherent in the mercurian process.

Chapter 9

Mercury in mythology

Manifestations of Mercury

In this chapter the terms Hermes and Mercury are interchangeable, both being established names (Greek and Roman respectively) for the messenger god. In Greek his name 'Hermes' also means 'interpreter', 'the word' and 'the logos or verbum'. Mercury spoke through the Greek oracles with messages such as:

"I am he whom you call the Son of the Father [Zeus] and Maia. Leaving the King of Heaven [the Sun] I come to help you, mortals".

Elsewhere he is depicted having three heads and called 'Tricephalos' or 'Triplex', and being one with the Sun and Venus. Mercury is known as the Hebrew Enoch, the Scandinavian Odin, the Christian Archangel Michael and the Mazdean Mithra who was a genius God placed between the Sun and the Moon (and depicted as the God of Wisdom). Mercury's wings symbolise his constant attendance on the Sun's course. He was also known as the Nuntius or Sunwolf. In Greek mythology he is depicted as one of the dogs (symbolising vigilance) watching over the celestial flock and the Argus watching over Earth.

Mythology of Gemini
In astrology, Mercury the planet has exoteric rulership over the zodiacal sign of Gemini. Esoteric rulership involves a change of rulership of the various planets within the solar system (see p.74).

The constellation Gemini contains the two bright stars Castor and Pollux, also called the twins, which throughout myth have been labelled the stars of duality. Although both were sons of Zeus, only Pollux was immortal, whilst Castor was a mere human mortal. They were however inseparable as brothers, such that Pollux begged Zeus to let him also die after Castor was killed in a contest. However immortal gods were not able to die, so Zeus ordained that Pollux spent half the year in the heavens with the other gods and the other half in the underworld with his brother. This is revealed in the constellations by the setting of Castor below the western horizon followed then by the setting of Pollux. Conversely, soon after the rise of Castor in the eastern horizon Pollux rises also.

The twins governed doorways and entrances, hence the symbol for Gemini as the two pillars. This is in keeping with Mercury's role as psychopomp, guiding souls through the entrance into the underworld and higher spiritual realms.

The works of Homer

Mercury features variously in the great works by Homer, the 'Illiad', 'Odyssey' and the 'Hymn' published in this order. Not much of his character is revealed in the 'Illiad'; more is found in the 'Odyssey'. Even more depth is revealed in the 'Hymn', where he features as a hero. This is not to say that Homer was not aware of these other qualities of Mercury, only that the level with which Mercury functions in each epic is in line with the developmental stage of humanity at the time. Thus Mercury is a peripheral character in the 'Illiad'; it is Achilles who dominates this story. However in this book the nature of the death process is shown by the daimon of fate (see p.93).

The birth of Mercury

Mercury is described as the son of Caelus and Lux (the sky and the light, or the Sun). He is also variously known as the progeny of Jupiter/Zeus and Maia. He becomes the messenger of his father Zeus, the Messiah of the Sun. Mercury was born on Mount Cyllene amongst shepherds, thus becoming their patron.

It is in Homer's 'Hymn' that Mercury is revealed in a heroic and more complete fashion. His birth origin is described:

'... whom Maia mothered, the nymph with beautiful hair, awesome, lying with Zeus. She kept away from the wonderful company of the gods, and lived in a shady cave. Here the son of Cronus [Zeus] had the nymph with beautiful hair, in the early hours of the evening, while sweet sleep held the pale arms of Hera, and where no man and no god could see.'

Instead of the usual Olympian goddesses, Mercury's mother Maia is a nymph, an Earth-spirit. She is bound up with Earth energies. Maia is also described as a daughter of the Titan Atlas, and also as one of the Pleiades, which suggest a Titaness. Thereby she is in effect one of the goddesses, but has shunned the immortal Olympian realm and taken abode in a cave on Earth. The love between Zeus and Maia is stolen love, for Zeus has secreted himself away from view – but for that it is all the more fully enjoyed. Zeus has deceived Hera through a sleep inducer. These factors interweave into the conception of Mercury and shape his future role. Thus it says of the pregnancy:

'... she produced her child, the very crafty, the super-subtle Hermes: thief, cattle-rustler, carrier of dreams, secret agent, prowler, and soon to show his stuff with the immortal gods.'

The number four in numerology represents Earth, and has a special significance for Mercury, for he is a master guide for the soul's journey through the myriad Earth realms. He therefore is as well suited to travelling within, through and on Earth as he is in the spiritual realms beyond Earth. His association with this number is revealed:

'Born in the morning, he played the lyre by afternoon, and by evening had stolen the cattle of the Archer Apollo – all on the fourth day of this month in which the lady Maia produced him.'

Note the fourth day of each month was not only held in reverence of Mercury, but also Aphrodite – with whom he has a special relationship (see pp.103, 191).

The god of travel

Mercury is also the god of roads and crossroads. His head in marble (known in Greek as 'Herms') was placed in posts at crossroads to help point the way. Herms also marked the boundaries of properties, graves and the entrance to homes. A pile of stones sometimes served as the Herm.

In Greek mythology he is traditionally shown wearing a wide brimmed travelling hat, which acts as protection against the sun's rays. This reflects the fact that the planet Mercury is never far away from the Sun. The hat is used to stabilise the neural pathways under stimulation by the particular information Mercury is relaying. The brain is actually quite plastic in the manner in which it triggers electrical conduction and chemical neurotransmitters along the selected nerve fibre pathways. After a particular signal has passed down the designated nerve pathway, that route is cleared in readiness for further fresh new signals. Such signals are the thoughts streaming from the spiritual realm under the influence of the soul-spirit. Mercury requires his hat in order to fixate the nerve impulses he needs to pass onto his recipients, otherwise fresh signals from the spiritual realm would too easily distort the message he is trying to carry. It is noteworthy the metal Mercury was used in fur hat making and resulted in many cases of poisoning of the hatters (see p. 143).

He fashioned winged sandals out of tamarisk and myrtle branches, this latter plant being related to death forces in the ancient world. He also travels without effort and his tracks are confusing and impossible to follow. In a sense he literally volatises in front of people's eyes like a breath of wind. Compare this with the volatility of metallic Mercury, which easily vaporises into gas.

MERCURY IN MYTHOLOGY

The caduceus

This is the wand or rod carried by Mercury (Fig. 9-1). It has two serpents or snakes twined upward around it. The upper part features either two small wings or a winged helmet.

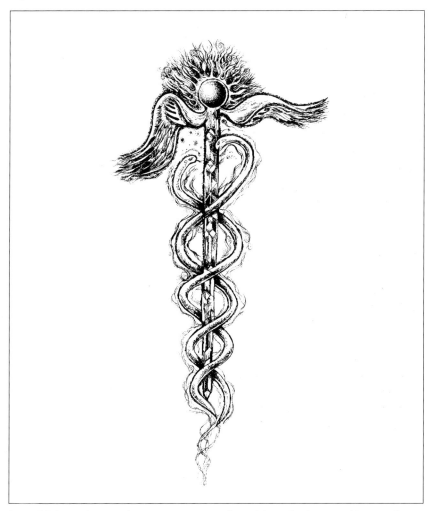

[Fig. 9.1] *Caduceus of Mercury. There are two serpents twined around the wand and surmounted by two small wings (or sometimes a winged helmet).*

83

The coiled snakes

The two coiled snakes have deep esoteric significance. There are many references in ancient spiritual treatises revealing that names of God are synonymous with the serpent that originally lured Adam and Eve into the material plane. In Sanskrit this is also the 'Dragon of Wisdom' and is the One, also known as 'Eka' or 'Saka'. Jehovah's name in Hebrew is also derived from One, 'Ehad'. The symbol for a dragon is the same as that for 'Astral Light' or 'Primordial Principle' or 'Wisdom of Chaos'.

Ancient philosophy did not focus on the duality of good or evil, but considered all as manifestations from the 'Absolute All' of universal perfection. Pure light condensed into matter or form and became depicted as evil polarised to the spiritual aspect of light. The word devil was also corrupted from the ancient wisdom of the Hindu Devas and the later Zoroastrians. In many cultures the snake has represented divine wisdom and perfection, and imbued psychical regeneration and immortality. Mercury stated that the snake was the most spiritual of all beings. The two snakes of the caduceus reveal the dual power of black and white magic. Through this was given the power to guide souls into the spiritual realm after physical death, but also the power to bring back life to the 'dead', as resurrection. Jesus Christ anchored these mercurial powers during his incarnation for this very purpose.

There are seven vowels depicted on the head of the snake in gnostic lore, which represent the seven hierarchies of the planetary creators. Before the Earth became physically manifest, a fiery dragon is described as moving in the infinitudes alone. Before even the universe came into being, a long trail of cosmic dust or fire-mist moved and writhed like a serpent in space. This was the Spirit of God moving chaos, and was symbolised in culture by a dragon breathing light and fire upon primordial waters, thus incubating cosmic matter. The serpent placed its tail inside its own mouth, assuming annular shape to represent the globes formed in space out of the fiery mist. The stars and planets were then cast off like old serpent skins, followed by periods of rest before the next cycle of creation.

The pranic tube

Energetically the staff is able to connect to the pranic tube of the soul. There is a column of light about 10 cm in diameter that connects the alpha and omega chakras together and runs along the spinal region of the body. The alpha chakra is an energy centre 15-20 cm above the head that interfaces with the totality and vastness of the spirit of the individual. This chakra conveys the immense amount of information coming to the incarnated soul from all the aspects of its spirit across spiritual reality and beyond time, space and incarnations. The omega chakra is 15-20 cm below the coccyx and interfaces with the rest of the soul's experiences across its incarnational grid. Thus it conveys into the soul all the experiences it has, is and will be acquiring across all time and space co-ordinates in material and subtle manifestation.

Essentially the column of light between alpha and omega conveys all that a soul is 'up there' to all that a soul is 'down here'. Within this column there is another tube, about 3-4 cm in diameter, called the pranic tube, which carries the specific frequencies of light and other energy required in the particular incarnation at hand. Three waveforms travel within this inner tube, also called the waves of Metatron (who is the King of the Archangels and responsible for all light in the universe). These are the electrical, magnetic and gravitational waves. The spinal cord of concentrated nervous tissue is simply the final material or densified manifestation of this pranic tube. For most souls there is debris and tainted energy within their pranic tube and consequently within their physical spinal cord. Most human personalities do not 'own their own spine', or could be called 'spineless' and 'without backbone'. All these phrases refer to the character trait of not being able to stand on one's own two feet, to take responsibility for one's actions, words and thoughts. Strength of character prevents others controlling the individual journey of one's own soul. This is not an aggressive stance; rather it is the ability to truly know oneself, without reference to any other being.

The staff of Mercury has the magical quality of revealing to the soul the clarity and purity of its own pranic tube. For less developed souls, fearful of death and fearful of the journey, the pranic tube invariably contains karmic issues incomplete from the incarnation just left behind. The soul is forced to take responsibility for its actions, it learns to judge itself with the help of Mercury and ancillary beings, but in doing so the staff can appear hideous and grisly. For those souls of pure heart and mind, the staff helps them align their pranic tube with the realms above and below the material Earth, and indeed invites them to activate the Mercury within themselves. The staff thus appears golden, with the required Christ mastery codes needed for the soul. Mercury symbolises the power of the journey itself, that in fact there is no definite start and stop point, no actual home for the soul on or off the Earth world. Rather the soul is made aware of its home as the path it walks, it learns to let go of all past memories and experiences and to not expect further events – but to simply let the journey unfold. The soul becomes open to all adventures and to all of nature. This is the state realised when the soul merges with the Mercury within, fulfilling the role of Mercury for Earth and releasing Mercury as the god from this obligation. Until then Mercury the god is constantly alongside the soul on the road, he is constantly in motion with the human souls. Even at rest, Mercury portrays a dynamic restlessness, an impulse to move onward.

The messenger of the gods

The scattering of souls
With the separation of humans souls from their formerly constant alignment with the spiritual realm the Earth world became fragmented into many 'mansion worlds', or worlds within worlds. These myriad dimensions of reality provided the human soul with infinite possibilities for soul growth through the journey of reincarnation. Only Mercury could provide the integrating quality for the human soul to understand the journey as a complete unity. Mercury provided the experience of forgetfulness and the veils of unconsciousness required for souls to properly deal with their experience at hand. Otherwise souls would be too bound to past experiences and the karma within

those 'past lives'. They would be too aware of the other possibilities available to them from supersensible realities. They would find it difficult in fact to stay in the relatively mundane slower third-dimensional material Earth plane. This is reflected in the ability of Mercury metal to scatter into myriad droplets, yet re-constitute once again completely into a single whole mass.

For this purpose Mercury is required to journey alongside humanity even to the depths of their lives inside the Earth. Mercury needs to be intimately linked to the Earth; his realm is not the higher realm of the other [Greek] gods, but closer to the Earth. He is also providing messages from the gods but without responsibility or obligation of the human soul, for otherwise the soul would not have a sense of free will or the ability to carve its own destiny on Earth. The mischievous and rebellious aspect of Mercury comes through in this regard. Whoever accepts the messages from Mercury must also be willing to lose out, as well as to profit or make gains. Mercury has a kind and gentle character flipping instantly into taking a delight at the misfortune of others. He energetically rules the life and death processes, the ability to take up as well as the ability to let go.

Here is revealed also the messenger role of Mercury when he imparts the message given to him from Zeus:

'No words were lost on Hermes the Wayfinder, who bent to tie his beautiful sandals on, ambrosial, golden, that carry him over water or over endless land in a swish of the wind, and took the wand with which he charms asleep – or when he wills, awakens – the eyes of men.'

Mercury is a master of taking oaths. His son, Autolycos, was also trained in such mastery. This is the power to hold a human soul responsible to the promises and destined fate it has agreed to during its incarnations. However the gift of cunning belongs also to Mercury and his descendants (one of whom was Odysseus), although after Autolycos it dissipated into mere versatility. Autolycos retained the power to shapeshift and to make invisible everything he touched.

Humanity's need for guidance
The mythology of Mercury during the time of ancient Greece needs to be understood from the perspective of human consciousness at the time, and before. Mythology is not some fantasy conjured up for storytelling or even for its symbolic meaning. The gods and other extraordinary beings were real and perceptible, when the veils of consciousness between the other realms and the material were not as densely separated as they are now. However early humanity had not yet developed the sense of ego or personal identity. Instead a tribal and group-oriented consciousness existed. Humanity felt bound up with the fates destined for them and was controlled or guided by supernatural beings, including the mythic gods. They felt the presence of angels, demons and nature spirits, who all played their part in the grand tapestry of Earth life. Humans felt the constant protection and guidance particularly of their guardian angel that helped maintain the stability of the physical-etheric vehicles between incarnations and between day-waking and night-sleeping cycles.

When Homer wrote the 'Illiad', 'Odyssey' and the 'Hymn', he had in mind the major developmental phases of the human consciousness and the influence of the gods. Mercury is a key player in understanding how the gods interacted with humans. To understand Mercury is to perceive meditatively the consciousness of this being behind the stories, behaviour, adventures and physical appearance. There is a definite energy and character that we can call the being Mercury and he has had many guises and many other names throughout mythology.

The Fates
In Homer's 'Hymn', Apollo is revealed bestowing upon Mercury a gift of divination by way of the Fates. Apollo is described saying:

'For there are some Fates, three of them, sisters by birth, virgins who take pleasure in their swift wings. Their heads have been sprinkled over with a white barley-powder. They make their homes under the cliffs of Parnassus. They taught divination independent of me, while I was still a child practising it around my cattle. My father didn't stop them. From there, they fly, now here, now there, and eat beeswax and accomplish everything. And when they have fed on the golden honey, they are inspired and want to pronounce truths, all of their own accord. If, however, they are kept away from this sweet food of the gods, then they try to lead you astray.'

This description is remarkably close to that of bees, which have swift wings, heads sprinkled with pollen (white barley-powder), feed on wax to make honeycombs and also on honey. The ancient Greeks considered bees to have souls, full of enthusiasm and having the power of prophecy. On another level, the Fates were three of the daughters of Zeus by his second wife Themis. They were called Clotho, Lachesis and Atropos, and collectively called the Fates for they determined the destiny of each individual human being.

This destiny was symbolised by a thread, which the first Fate drew from her distaff, the second wound up and the third Fate cut when the span of life was completed. There is an esoteric relationship between bees and the Fates. Bees live completely by the laws of the Sun, indeed they are sunlight in animal form. They are part of the stream of energy by which the sun travels from flower to pollen to bee and thence to honey. Indeed honey even gives the appearance of liquid sunlight.

The consciousness being ensouling the Sun of our solar system is Helios, a masculine consciousness. Astrologically Helios carries within its being the blueprints defining the destiny of all human souls working through the Earth school. The future of each human is stored within the core of the Sun. The Sun is also a stargate or dimensional doorway for reception and transmission of new life purpose and destiny when a human spiritual seeker connects to far flung universal and cosmic consciousness. Thus Mercury has an important relationship with Helios the Sun, assisting the conveyance of information regarding destiny. The Fates are part of this Hermetic team effort. Mercury has a deep respect for the judgements of the Fates, no matter how frivolous he may appear in myth, for he must honour the individual destiny chosen by each human soul. His role is not to disrupt the thread of life purpose but to facilitate it.

The ibis form of Thoth
The consciousness beings or deities that represent solar (Sun) and lunar (Moon) energy have frequently throughout history been depicted by the symbol of birds. The ibis bird is sacred to Isis, whose head often assumes its form (Fig. 9.2). Similarly so for Mercury who as Thoth adopted the form of an ibis to escape from Typhon. This latter being was one of the fallen angels and aligned to the Kabeira (see p.112) and also depicted as the god Seth by the ancient Semites, especially in Palestine and ancient Egypt. The ibis was a venerated bird in Egypt. There were however two kinds of ibis, one fully black, the other black and white. The black type was fiercer and was said to prevent infestation of Egypt from winged serpents coming from Arabia each winter. The other anchored the energy of the Moon, being as white and brilliant as its lit side, and also dark like its shadow side. The ibis could kill land serpents and destroy the eggs of crocodiles, thus limiting excessive infestation of the Nile by these creatures. It was said the ibis would be most active and powerful in this regard under moonlight. Thoth guided the ancient Egyptians in the form of an ibis, teaching them secrets of the occult. The ibis, amongst other powerful birds such as the albatross and white swan, was a vehicle for such magical powers.

Divination was also made possible through the use of sacred birds. The technique of oomancy is especially relevant, taught by the underworld god Orpheus. Under certain conditions, studying the yolk and white of a bird's egg would reveal all that the bird would actually come to see during its coming life. This was an ancient learned art, but has since degenerated into a cheap fortune-teller's trick.

The ibis as represented by Thoth imparts the quality Mercury needs to maintain the truth and wisdom behind the message he conveys from the spiritual realm to humanity. It is the nature of earthly incarnation to be uncertain about the future outcome of any action within the material plane. If humanity retained the same accurate spiritual and psychic

MERCURY IN MYTHOLOGY

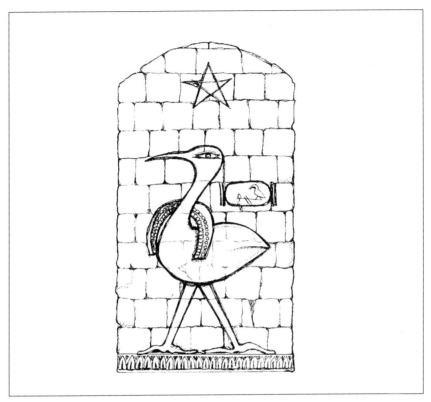

[Fig. 9.2] *Ibis form of Thoth.*

cognisance in the material plane, as they possess within the spiritual plane, then nothing would actually be a challenge. A human would always know the best approach to take in all matters, and truly never make a 'mistake'. But discovery, exploration and learning require the soul to enter a state of relative illusion and unconsciousness during its earthly incarnations.

However too great a rift between the incarnated personality and its spirit creates difficulty, such as personality fragmentation, excessive confusion, delirium or hallucination. Schizoid states of personality can arise. If the message conveyed to humans under the guidance of Mercury were to become too misaligned from the actual truth in the spiritual realm, then humans would fall into mental madness. This explains the disordered mental states in the picture of homoeopathic Mercury (see p.7). The bird symbol of Mercury as Thoth reveals the fact that the essence behind his message is truth and wisdom, even if this is not at first apparent to the receiving human personality. In mythology Mercury is known as the Lord of Wisdom. A quote by Vossius is revealing:

'All the theologians agree to say that Mercury and the Sun are one... He was the most eloquent and the most wise of all the Gods, which is not to be wondered at, since Mercury is in such close proximity to the Wisdom and the Word of God [the Sun] that he was confused with both.'

The death process

In the formation of the human, the Earth supplies the body, the Moon the animal soul, and the Sun the ego clothed in abstract mental substance. When this composition returns to the spiritual worlds at death there is effectively a double death. First the animal soul is separated from the body, and the mythological beings assisting this include Demeter and earthly Mercury (as the lord of souls). This animal soul undergoes a certain amount of penance in the middle sphere in order to purify it of animalistic tendencies, and is caught up in the Moon to pass through the Earth's shadow during an eclipse. Those with much negativity to clear are not allowed to enter a paradise state, being frightened away from this by seeing a 'terrible face'.

On the other hand, good souls enjoy tranquillity in the Moon's sphere, and assist earthly affairs, enjoying being of service. After a certain time the soul desires to ascend further into the sphere of the Sun, and the ego/mental body is extracted from the animal soul, with the assistance of Persephone and celestial Mercury, in a gentle fashion. This is the second death. The liberated soul flies upward to merge with universal life force. Meanwhile the animal soul that is left continues a dreamy sort of life in the Moon sphere, to be gradually dissolved rather like the decomposition of the physical body back on Earth. Calm and philosophic souls, for whom reason has overcome emotions, are easily absorbed into the lunar field. Active and passionate animal souls are more difficult to dissipate, and continue to wander about within the middle sphere. The Moon is the mother of generations, and rules over mists and vapours.

The physical body is composed of five elements, and the animal soul composed of seven elements, the ego/mental body of twelve elements.

When the ego/mental body casts off the animal soul to return to the Sun sphere, it must escape through seven gates, for the animal soul is built out of seven elements or colours. A planet rules each of these seven. If the ego has knowledge it can elude these seven planetary powers to ascend into the eighth heaven, that of the Universal Mother. These seven planets have even been seen as the lords of death, for they weave the tangled webs of destiny that bond the ego to the inferior world. There are words of power that when uttered will allow the soul to overcome these binds during the death process, and indeed overcome the whole death process to become immortal. During this process it can be realised that the head and brain is a mirror for the whole cosmos.

The daimon of fate

In the 'Illiad', Mercury (as Hermes) portrays the gaseous phase of Mercury the metal; he is not in a definite enough material form to guide human souls along individualised journeys. Human souls needed to sufficiently individualise for this to occur, and part of this process required a guardian angel and daimon of fate to incorporate into each human soul matrix. Achilles undergoes such an intertwining. After being anointed upon birth by his mother, his remaining weak point is the achilles tendon. From the beginning we realise his fate, that of death, is stamped on his frame. He is not tricked by death as some luring process, nor is it an unfamiliar process – for he is living with death inside him throughout his life. Death is inescapable and no amount of complaint will remove the finality and law of this for him.

His daimon of fate enters his soul upon his physical birth, and ripens into a daimon of death. This daimon is in truth the suffering aspect of his human soul, as it journeys through youth and manhood to a dark death. It has individualised his incarnational journey like no other process, for inherent laws become embedded into the soul matrix through the daimon. Mercury does not here have any role as escort or guide for the soul after death, for human souls were not yet fully integrated with their personalised daimon of death to understand and perceive the underworld realities of the journey after death. Until then souls had more or less retained a sense of group awareness even after death, thus not realising they were each on a personal journey and not meant to be sharing or merging their paths with each other in some herd like fashion.

Mercury therefore functions outwith the physical Earth world, where death is the backdrop to material reality, the alternative to life on Earth. In the 'Illiad', Mercury is almost resolutely staying away from any role as guide for souls, he is not a messenger god at this point, and is not even himself portrayed as a hero-god. He does not seek fame. For example he evades having to fight with his assigned opponent Leto, the mother-goddess of Artemis, saying:

'since it is a hard thing to come to blows with the brides of Zeus who gather the clouds. No sooner you may freely speak among the immortal Gods, and claim that you were stronger than I, and beat me.'

Thoth and ancient Egypt

Mercury could weigh the dead soul as part of the judgement required. Thoth incarnated as Mercury for the purpose of developing the post-Atlantean civilisations (in South America, Egypt, India, China, Britain, etc.) and was the record keeper in Egypt. Thoth assisted the weighing of the human soul soon after it left its physical incarnation, for the purpose of planning the next phase of the journey into heaven or into hell.

This role has been depicted in the Hall of Judgement in 'The Egyptian Book of the Dead' – where he is ibis-headed and standing next to a pair of scales or a pivot. He is there measuring with a ruler the weight of the soul, represented by the heart of the newly dead, relaying this to Osiris, god of the dead and of resurrection. Osirus is equivalent to the greek god Hades. Anubis is the dog-headed god in charge of the actual physical weighing (Fig. 9-3). The heart is counterbalanced on measuring scales by a feather, which belongs to Ma-a-t, the goddess of

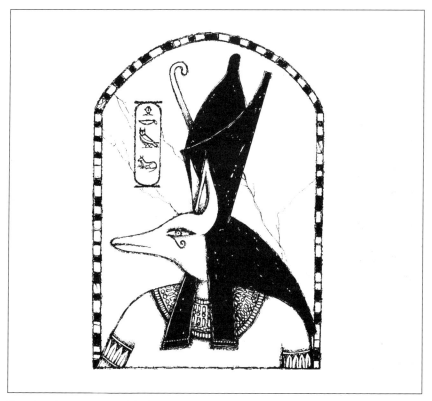

[Fig. 9.3] *Anubis, an incarnation of Thoth.*

truth and justice. The weighing also measures the balance of Moon and Sun forces within the soul, which represent the forces of its past and future biography, pulling it into each direction within the astral plane.

Guide to the dead souls, the psychopomp
Later in Homer's epics, Mercury as the psychopomp conducts dead souls to the underworld. Sometimes he would guide a soul back to Earth, as in the case of Persephone. His magic staff with the caduceus helped him pave the journey. Mercury collaborated with the many denizens of the underworld. These included the demon Tuchulcha, the guide Charon, underworld gods such as Orcus (another death god) and Libitina (goddess of funerals), and the Lemunes or Larvae who were ghosts of the dead returned to the surface world to torment the living.

In the 'Odyssey', Mercury reveals his true skills in 'summoning up' the soul out of its physical body prior to burial or body destruction and leading them onward to the next phase of the journey. Through his staff he can lull souls to sleep and re-awaken them in a different form. Death in the 'Odyssey' is not portrayed as a final end, but a doorway to the next reality. In the last book of the 'Odyssey' we have:

'Meanwhile the suitors' ghosts were called away by Hermes of Kyllene, bearing the golden wand with which he charms the eyes of men or wakens whom he will. He waved them on, all squeaking as bats will in a cavern's underworld, all flitting, flitting criss-cross in the dark if one falls and the rock-hung chain is broken. So with faint cries the shades trailed after Hermes, pure deliverer. He led them down dank ways, over gray Ocean tides, the Snowy Rock past shores of Dream and narrows of the sunset, in swift flight to where the Dead inhabit wastes of asphodel at the world's end.'

A word that also describes Mercury is 'eriounios', which can translate as 'the quick one' and is also used to describe gods who receive human sacrifices. Mercury here is as 'fast as death'; he is the death god. The staff of Mercury is depicted as golden and beautiful, creating a distance between the god and the dark swarm of bat-souls. However at times it is depicted (usually from the perspective of fearful souls about to enter the death-journey) as a horrid wand:

'His grisly wand let Hermes once uphold, the blood returns not to the formless shade. The sable company he troops below, in idle ears against their doom appeal.'

The golden aspect of the staff is revealed in:

'Thou layest unspotted souls to rest; thy golden rod pale spectres know; Blest power! By all thy brethren blest, above, below.'

Thus does Mercury appear gentle and kind even to the unfortunate souls in the underworld, where he is also named 'akaketa' or 'painless' for his ability to soften their suffering. The staff reveals a vital power of Mercury – for he has the ability to show to the human soul the lessons it must complete on the phase of the journey at hand. This not as some objective and judgmental God, but in his capacity to reveal what is hidden within the soul itself.

Hades the underworld

In the Odyssey, Apollo describes another aspect of Mercury's messenger role:

'...it's for the glorious Hermes to rule, and to be the only recognised messenger to Hades, who himself never takes a gift from anybody. This time, though, he will give him a gift that is far from least.'

The text implies this role is only recognised after Mercury undergoes a preliminary ceremony or initiation. It was frequently said that a friendly relationship with Hades could only come about through a death-oriented initiation, and was part of the teachings of the Kabeirean Mysteries (a secret order, see p.111). This involved an understanding by Mercury of the rules of the underworld and with it the ability to penetrate into the subconscious realm of humanity. The underworld is governed, or to be more correct, administered by Hades on behalf of humanity. During the journey karmic cords invariably exist between souls especially at the level of the abdominal chakras. These cords maintain ties between souls, which define their journey after death of the physical body. Many elemental beings supervise these karmic inter-relationships, which have often been depicted as demons in hell. In truth hell is a human construct, it is a realm of illusion created by human souls to trap soul fragments caught in such underworld karmic ties. The experience of hell is perceived as real by the soul fragment, until it realises it has the key to its own salvation and can then undergo the process of redemption and resurrection. The soul fragment can then leave the underworld of hell and return to the rest of its soul in the overworlds or spiritual realm.

Mercury has a key role in guiding the soul (or its fragment) into the underworld of Hades so as to experience its illusionary karmic entrapment – invariably with pain and suffering. It is not Mercury's role to save the human soul, and his initiation into Hades taught him to respect the individual journey of the soul. If Mercury were to interfere and change the path of the soul rather than simply guide it along the destined path, then he would have had to share in the karmic suffering. Nevertheless Mercury is described as a creature of the night, and inflicts many deceptions on humanity:

'And that's how the Lord Apollo came to love the son of Maia, with many signs of friendship, and the son of Cronus [Zeus] added his favor. And Hermes mingles now with all men and gods. And even though he helps a few people, he cheats an endless number of the race of mortal men in the darkness of the night.'

However this is only deception of humanity at the level of materialistic duality. From the higher perspective of the human spirit, Mercury guides the soul through the initiation of death through the letting go of the material roles, possessions and memories the soul had of its physical incarnation on Earth. In so doing the soul is loosened or no longer bound to its former incarnation, liberating it to continue its journey into kamaloka and devachen (the stages between earthly lives) and onto the next incarnation. Without Mercury human souls would become trapped into a cycle of perpetual memories, roles and relationships.

Ruler of thieves and liars

With this role he shows the most unheroic evasiveness in his behaviour. Mercury is the master thief and liar as shown in the 'Illiad'. He is illustrated as handsome, friendly, yet also deceitful and thievish. With his magical golden shoes he travels around the Earth and seas, and is able to induce sleep in people through his golden staff. He reveals the early signs here as a seductive guide of souls, with the power of death available to him.

Thus he crept out of the cave that was his birth home, and sought the cattle herd tended by his elder brother Apollo. Whilst Apollo's attentions were elsewhere, Mercury stole the herd and cleverly walked backwards to confuse anyone following his tracks. He returned to his cave and climbed quietly into his cot, but his mother couldn't be fooled and questioned him. Apollo eventually arrived and suspected Mercury of the theft, but could find no evidence in the cave. Mercury meanwhile pretended to be a sleeping baby, holding his lyre under his arm. However Apollo recognised Mercury as a son of Zeus, and said to him:

"Listen kid, lying in your cradle, tell me where my cows are, and quick! We're going to fight this out and it won't be very pretty! I'm going to take you and throw you into black Tartarus, into a hopeless darkness. What a terrible end! And neither your mother nor your father will bring you back to the light of day! You'll wander upon the earth, leading little people around!"

Little people here refers to the dead souls wandering around in the underworld and is an allusion to the role of Mercury as psychopomp or guide for dead souls. Apollo threatens him with confinement in that realm. Mercury's reply to his brother is a classic illustration of his deviousness and ability to lie, and yet retain a sense of humour:

"Son of Leto, why do you speak so rudely, and why come here looking for your animals? I didn't see anything, I didn't learn anything, I didn't hear anything from anybody else. I don't have any information to give, and the reward for information wouldn't go to me if I did. I'm not like a person who drives away cattle, I'm not big enough! This wasn't my work! I'm interested in other kinds of things: sleep is what I care about, and the milk of my mother. I care about blankets around my shoulders. And having hot baths! I sure hope nobody hears what this argument is about!

And it would be a surprise for the gods: a baby just new-born, who could walk right in the door with a herd of cows. What you're talking about is ridiculous. I was born yesterday! My feet are still pretty soft. The ground underneath is pretty hard. If you want, I'll swear a great oath on the head of my father: I declare that I am myself not guilty, nor did I see any other thief of your cattle, whatever cattle are, anyway – I've only heard of them."

And while he said this, he peeked out from under his bright eyelids, looking here and there. And he whistled too, for a long time, like somebody listening to a lie. Apollo, laughing softly, said to him:

"You trickster, you sharpie, the way you talk I bet you have broken into a lot of expensive homes in nights past and left more than one man with nothing more to sit on than his doorsill, looting his home without a sound. And you'll be a nuisance to shepherds in the fields of mountain-valleys, whenever you're in the mood for meat, and you come across herds of cattle and flocks of sheep. But come on, get out of that cradle, unless you want to sleep your deepest and final sleep, come on, companion of black night! For from now on you will hold this honor among the gods: for all time you will be called The Prince of Thieves!"

Phoebus Apollo said this and then seized him. The powerful Argeiphontes lifted up by the god's arms intentionally released an omen, an insolent servant of his stomach, a reckless little messenger. Right after this he suddenly sneezed too.'

Thus Mercury shows his indecent nature through releasing a stool in front of the clean god Apollo. Mercury also repeats his untruthful oath in front of Zeus, and both Apollo and Zeus laugh at his perjury. In the event, Apollo accepts the lyre in return for Mercury keeping the cattle. Mercury becomes patron of shepherds and cattle herders, obtaining a staff to function as a whip. The power of oracle and prediction is also divided up between the two godly brothers. Apollo retains the power of secret counsel, of what 'lies in the mind of Zeus alone', with which he can help or punish humans. Mercury is not to be trusted with such power, and is treated by Apollo not as his equal but as 'Daimon of the Gods'. This function is not as a detached divine being, but as intermediary with the mortal realm, one who reveals or heralds the truth and is swift as death. This equates to the role of Apollo in his capacity as Helios, the solar logos, to hold the codes for the future destiny of human souls evolving through Earth. Mercury functions as the intermediary between these Sun and Earth realms.

Ruler of discovering and finding

Upon his birth, Mercury straightaway reveals his rushing and quick nature, the 'Hymn' literally describes him leaping out of the cradle:

'For after he jumped down from the immortal loins of his mother he couldn't lie still very long in his sacred cradle, but leaped right up to search for the cattle of Apollo, climbing over the threshold of this high-roofed cave.'

Furthermore,

'There he found a turtle and it brought him lots of fun: Hermes was the first to manufacture songs from the turtle he encountered outside the door, as it was eating the splendid grass...'

Part of Mercury's nature is to constantly meet and find things of use and of revelation. He also takes endless delight in such experiences, for Mercury there is always something of great fortune (or misfortune depending on who's perspective) in finding things in the material realm, for he can perceive their divine purpose and message. He epitomises the quality of accidental discovery, which has been called a hermetical activity by the alchemists. Mercury is also a master of appropriating such 'finds' when they actually belong to the realm of the gods, for example through theft he puts objects to better use. Indeed the Greek word for windfall is 'Hermaion', belonging thus to Hermes. This was also the name given to offerings to the gods left at roadsides, but 'stolen' by travellers. By ruling over thieves, Mercury declares his approval of seizing accidental finds and claiming them as one's own. This quality within commercial and business dealings is also governed by Mercury, where a trader enters the middle territory between the respective parties and appropriates that which is most advantageous to him/her. It is not an immoral unscrupulous energy that Mercury holds with respect to theft, but the intelligent art of living. Indeed Hercules governs the stupid witless people who benefit through fortune and windfall, for they often continue to make stupid mistakes rather than develop new creative impulses from the experience.

With regards to the turtle, the story continues:

'The son of Zeus, the helper, looked at it, then burst out laughing, and said this:

"What a great sign, what a help this is for me! I won't ignore it. Hello there, little creature, dancing up and down, companion at festivals, how exciting it is to see you. Where did your beautiful covering come from? Your shell is kaleidoscopic, you're a turtle which lives in the mountains. But I'm going to pick you up and take you home with me. You'll be a big help to me, and I won't slight you, but you have to help me first. You'll find it much better at our house – outside here things are bad. Alive, of course, you're good medicine against the pains of black magic. But dead, dead you'll make great music!"

He said all this, then, picking up this lovable toy with both hands he returned to his house, carrying it with him. When he got back he took out a grey, steel knife and stabbed out the life of the turtle that lived in the mountains.'

Here Mercury shows his hermetic quality of being able to see through objects, to perceive their divine purpose. He sees through the living turtle shell and perceives its capacity to make music. He already calls it 'friend of the feast', seeing its future role as background music through the lyre for such occasions. He sees this glorious role whilst the turtle is still alive. He then reveals his ability to activate a swift death and this in a merciless yet joyful mood. Consequently the music he plays has the capacity to induce sleep and even death for those who listen.

Music and Venus

Continuing the story from Homer's 'Hymn':

'And when it was finished, he took up the lovely toy and tried it out with a pick. It sounded terrible! The god tried to improvise, singing along beautifully, as teen-age boys do, mockingly at festivals, making their smart cracks.'

The relationship between Mercury and music is further understood when the ancient history of Venus is noted. (For a full coverage consult the Venus/Copper book in this series.) The early civilisations on planet Venus were a very musically gifted race. Indeed they formulated a caste system whereby the most skilled musicians and singers were accorded the highest status, followed by musical instrument makers and patrons of music. Lower down were the merchant and administrative class of workers. The manual workers without the same refined musical gifts were the lowest caste. However the Venusian nature was very sexually oriented, and much promiscuous intercourse between them led to genetically mutated individuals, particularly from incestuous coupling. Venusians are naturally very beautiful looking people, thus they felt shame and loathing towards these mutants amongst them. Much later in the course of their evolution there was a great deal of genetic research in an attempt to remove the mutant genes from their gene pool.

One of the early impulses for incorporating biological life on Earth was for reptilian Venusian genes to be embedded into the 'clay' of Earth –

a reference to the mineral Earth substance used to provide base substrate for the genetic code of the human race. Reptile energy is a very powerful tool to link genetic information to the subconscious and primordial depths of a planet. Another clue to this tale is that music and sound is a key energy used to shape the genetic code. Various mantras or words of power can be used meditatively to restructure the genetic code, tools which future medicine will discover. Mercury therefore needed a reptilian source of material (i.e. a turtle shell) with which to anchor the ancient Venusian musical gifts down to Earth.

It is interesting to consider the content of the songs of Mercury, for he knew no shame and sang insolently of the love affair between his parents.

'He sang about Zeus, the son of Cronos, and Maia in her beautiful shoes, how they talked during their love affair, a boast about his own glorious origin. And he honoured the servants of the nymph and her magnificent house. And the tripods in the house. And the abundant cauldrons.'

This is shameless when compared with the songs by others referring to the love affairs between the gods and other beings. Usually a song would simply refer to when and where the love affair takes place; it is however considered improper to go into details. This example of the shamelessness of Mercury is essentially a description of the phallic essence of Zeus his father. It also reveals that quality of Mercury that is conscious of his own origins and his ability to channel ancient Saturn energies on behalf of others (required for recall of past lives during the soul's journey). It reveals his willingness to make bold converse with the gods; he is not prudish and has no literary restraint. His ability to perceive the genealogy of the gods is revealed thus:

' Suddenly he started playing the lyre louder, reciting a prelude – and the sound accompanying him was lovely – about the immortal gods and the dark Earth, how they were in the beginning, and what prerogatives each one had. And the first of the gods that he commemorated with his song was Mnemosyne, Mother of Muses, for the son of Maia was a follower of hers. And all of them, all the immortal gods, according to age and how each one was born, the glorious son of Zeus recited, singing them all in order, playing his lyre on his arm.'

Mercury begins this song by going back to a source goddess, Mnemosyne, one of the ancient wives of Zeus. From her sprang many goddesses. She holds cosmic memory but also has the power to induce memory lapses. Along with Saturn (or Cronos/Chronos) she would provide the backdrop of cosmic memory out of which information Mercury can safely guide human souls along their path. In the Hymn, she is referred to as the daimon of fate set over Mercury. Mercury can thus never lose his anchor in cosmic memory, he can never himself forget – amongst other subjects he is possessed of the primordial history of the human race.

Mercury in myth and language

He was also associated with the number four and the shapes of the cross and the cube. This related to rulership over the faculty of speech. This was the word that includes all, the creative word or word of God as the seminal power throughout creation. This resonates with the philosophers Mercury within alchemy, as the principle holding the seed of the universe, fecundated by the solar fires.

Mercury (Hermes) is regarded as the inventor of language. The word 'herma' forms the basic root for the word 'hermeneia' meaning 'explanation'. Hermes is also 'hermeneus' or the 'interpreter'. He clarifies and is the God of Exposition.

Mercury and sexuality in myth

Of relevance here also is the god Eros, who is Mercury-like and rules over adventurers, lovers and sex. He is also known as the first masculine being in the cosmos, and is winged and as swift as the swift as death Mercury. Also, like Mercury, his nature is depicted as phallus, soul and spirit all at once. However he tends to be more idealistic a character than Mercury, as well as more binding and committed in his sexuality and relationships. In some myths, the first Eros was the son of Mercury with the first Artemis, and the second Eros the son of Mercury and the second Aphrodite. Mercury is shown as the phallic masculine principle aroused by the feminine.

Mercury is also known as lover of the nymphs, who are neither goddesses nor mortal women and are not immortal. The nymphs were mothers of the tree spirits. In these love sessions Mercury is often depicted as sharing the nymphs with the Silenoi, who are half-animal and very phallic creatures. The main Silenoi is Silenos, the phallic half-animal being who was the teacher of Dionysus, the god of the vineyard and wine. However Mercury is also often depicted as carrying the baby Dionysus on his arm, being the official bearer and guide for all divine children brought into the world. In this and other respects Mercury and Silenos are aspects of the same being. The divine-spiritual meets the divine-animal in friendly union.

Mercury is also assigned as permanent escort to the goddesses, who are often revealed as groups of three on countless reliefs in the Greek caves and hills. Here is revealed the essential trinity nature of the goddess – as primal mother, then daughter-bride and finally the warrioress/temptress.

Originally however the androgynous first being was known as Hermaphroditos and ascribed as the child of Mercury (Hermes) and Aphrodite. It was also said that Aphrodite was indeed the feminine aspect within Mercury, and conversely Mercury the masculine aspect within Aphrodite. The split into the two beings came about through arousal of the feminine and masculine natures. The realm for this separation or becoming was the primal water. Indeed Mercury was said to have possessed a spring containing sacred fish. He is equated with swamps, fishponds and springs. The great goddess in the form of Hecate was said to alternate between Mercury and the merman Triton for lovers. These associations with water and fish reveal the role Mercury played in the differentiation of humanity into male and female forms in ancient Lemuria, from androgynous fish-like primal creatures (see p.186).

Part of the soul's journey must involve combining the inner Mercury and Aphrodite through the integration of inner male and female energies. At that point the sacral chakra, which governs sexual energy and function, is properly aligned and integrates with the brow chakra. The human then has no need to externalise his/her inner gender problems through outer relationship issues. In any sexual relationship the personality can then truly honour the other partner, without sexual, emotional or psychic dependency on their partner. This activates male and female parts of the brain and endocrine system, especially at the pineal gland (which is male oriented) and the pituitary gland (which is feminine oriented). An inner sacred union of energy between these two glands occurs at the 'high altar' of the hypothalamic gland, and a subtle previously closed channel opens between the two through which flows cerebrospinal fluid. Mercury rules the activation of the masculine brain energies, and Aphrodite the activation of the feminine energies. The soul can then become the divine Hermaphrodite, i.e. having both male and female parts, not in the physical sense but within the subtle bodies.

The number three is also associated with Mercury, for he thereby assists the integration of divine male and female energies into the triplicity that is God — creating the third aspect of the soul which is hermaphrodite, Christed and the child aspect of God. His staff is thus three-pointed.

Asclepius and the Greco-Roman temples of healing

Asclepius is the Greek and Roman god of healing and medicine. His role involves several other gods, including Mercury (although Apollo has the greater role of the two). There are many references to Asclepius within Greek and Roman literature that has led scholars to suggest he was a real physician and renowned healer, but later elevated to a status of demi-god.

Asclepias was the child of a love affair between Apollo and Coronis of Larissa. However, when he heard of her infidelity, Apollo struck an arrow into her bosom, killing her. She was pregnant with their child at the time. Apollo was grief-struck upon coming to his senses and could not revive her despite his powerful healing techniques. Just before her body was consumed in the funeral pyre he rescued the child out of her womb. He passed the child onto Chiron, the centaur, who educated Asclepius in the arts of medicine. His birth was perfect for Asclepius to be able to channel the healing energies of Apollo, Mercury and the other gods. He carried the forces of the death initiation as well as resurrection into life within him. Death is a portal from the earthly material into the divine spiritual realm – and through this open connection Asclepius could even resurrect the dead. This, however, eventually incurred Zeus' wrath; who struck Asclepius with one of his lightning bolts in order to stop him.

The physicians of ancient Greece were known as Asclepiads, which literally means the 'offspring of Asclepias'. The best known was Hippocrates, who is accepted as the father of modern medicine today and taught the concept of imbalances between the four humours (black bile, yellow bile, phlegm and blood) underlying disease. Much of this knowledge continues to influence modern allopathic and complementary medical thought, often using different terms for largely the same vital energy. The practice of the Asclepiad included use of snakes as a means to access the subconscious and stimulate re-birth and regeneration. Asclepias carried a caduceus with a single coiled snake (see p.84). Indeed snakes had guarded the infant Asclepias on Mount Pelion and taught him the magical properties of herbs. He was also known to be able to shape-shift into a snake when needed.

Healing was mostly temple based, this being known as the Asclepieion. Such temples were built at scenes of great natural beauty with local healing springs. Included in the complex were bathing chambers (also for hydrotherapy), gymnasia, theatre, prayer chambers, meeting halls and incubation or sleep chambers. Mind-therapy was also given, which involved priest-physicians with special gifts for altering the mental state of patients and priest assistants who recanted the sacred words and held the sacred fires. This form of psychological conditioning has also been called nootherapy. Priests would pray for Asclepias to awaken from slumber and administer his healing on the patient.

The peak moment of the healing regimen for patients was the incubation, or ritual temple sleep treatment. They would usually receive the above treatments beforehand, especially nootherapy. The incubation was held within a special section of the temple known as the abaton. Entry was forbidden to those without permission or if the preliminary purification rituals had not been completed (which included ritual bathing in cold water). Patients slept in white garments and consumed special cakes flavoured with honey and wine as well as various potions to aid sleep. The sleep room, which contained a large statue of Asclepias, was lit with candles to maintain it in semi-darkness. As the patients slept the priests would walk amongst them with their dogs and snakes, allowing these creatures to periodically nudge and lick the patients.

The experience for each patient was unique and invariably they dreamt of the god Asclepias appearing and providing a healing. Generally, in the initial part of the dream, the god would make a diagnosis, often by placing his hand over the diseased part of their body. The treatment would consist of either a psychic surgical procedure, administering a mixture of herbs and animal parts, or advising the patient on some change in lifestyle or diet. For example the following case is recorded in the 'Inscriptiones Graecae' (which can be found in the 'Edelstein Testimonies', see Bibliography) and shows Asclepias curing a probable case of heart and lung failure (with lymphatic and fluid congestion or dropsy):

'Arata, a woman of Lacedaemon (Sparta), was dropsical. While she remained in Lacedaemon, her mother slept in the temple on her behalf and saw a dream. It seemed to her that the god cut off her daughter's head and hung up her body in such a way that her throat was turned downwards. Out of it came a huge amount of fluid. He then took down the body and fitted her head back onto her neck. After she had seen this dream she went back to Lacedaemon where she found her daughter in good health; she had seen the same dream.'

Asclepias often used parts of snakes in the concoctions, as well as ash of particular animals or plants. The following remedy was reported by Elder Pliny in his 'Natural History':

'The most effective remedies for diseases of the rectum are wool-grease...the ashes of a dog's head; the sloughed skin of a serpent, with vinegar. In cases where there is chapping, the ashes of the white portions of dogs' excreta, mixed with oil of roses; they say that this is an invention of Asclepias and that by the same treatment warts are most easily removed.'

Upon waking, patients would recall their dreams to the priests, who could offer explanations and further recommendations. Many were the cures reported from temple incubations, often with spectacular changes in the pathology of disease.

The benefit of sleep therapy derived more than from simply resting and recuperation. Modern scholars have generally assumed that the minor disturbance by the priests, dogs and snakes during the sleep would simulate dream experiences in the patients. However a visitation by the gods did occur. During sleep the gods had an opportunity to more directly communicate to the soul of the patient – ultimately for the purpose of strengthening the tie between the soul and body. Separation between the spiritual body (as vehicle for the soul) and the physical body underlies all disease. Most of humanity was still at an early stage of mental body development and lived more through their senses than their thoughts. During deep sleep the soul is normally freed from the physical body and travels to far-flung cosmic worlds. This indeed was the original reason for the need to sleep to become programmed into human consciousness. Without sleep it was probable that many souls would become too bound to the material realm and thus forget their spiritual origin, eventually leading to states of severe weariness and depression for earthly life. Through sleep the soul can receive new and fresh insights from the spiritual realm, to awaken rejuvenated and revitalised when returning to its body in the morning. However (due to the poor bond between the soul and its physical body), for most of humanity there are angels and spiritual guides that assist in rejuvenating the physical and etheric bodies in readiness for the morning re-incarnation of the soul. These beings are also known as guardians of the threshold. By way of soul healing during sleep the gods could repair damage in the soul and body linkage, as well as to develop the lower personality to accept greater levels of soul awareness during the day.

The incubation was effectively a form of initiation for soul-spiritual development. Mercury played a key role as one of the gods channelling through Asclepias, being able to guide the soul through the spiritual landscape between its physical body incarnations and retrieve stuck fragments of the soul in alternate realms of experience. Mercury could also assist the soul to selectively forget its past experiences, leading to cure of disease stemming from such aetiology (see p.115). Sleep therapy is indeed in its infancy of development, and souls now need to open up to further possibilities during deep sleep (the stages between rapid eye movement dreaming periods). Dreams, in the patient as well as the doctor, are themselves a fertile source of information for diagnostic and therapeutic purposes to the practitioner. The need now is for souls to strengthen the tie with the physical body through their own forces, rather than rely on the angels and gods for support of their body during the soul's exit. This is a rewarding area of spiritual research.

Kabeirean Mysteries and the fallen angels

The Kabira were descended Angels of Genesis and often depicted as divine priest kings. They entered the Earth sphere through the portals of Mercury and Venus during pre-Lemurian stages of Earth's evolution.

The role of the fallen angels included the need to instruct and guide early humans during their incarnations in such matters as agriculture, technology, astrology and health. Examples abound in stories around the world of gods and other higher beings appearing before humanity to impart some wisdom. Some have been depicted as acting out of compassion and sympathy for the human plight when separated from the spiritual realm. Thus Prometheus attempted to assist through the gift of fire – for which his fellow gods punished him. Some were ascended disciples and masters who chose to incarnate again into human society (even though they had gained liberation from the wheel of rebirth) in order to help their fellow humans in the ascension journey.

Another role for the fallen angels was incorporating their DNA within the human gene pool, providing much needed information for the further development of the human form along the divine blueprint. The divine image of the human as a god in the making is called Adam Kadmon (which incorporates both male and female forms, being the true hermaphrodite with sacred union of all polarities). However many fallen angels have also been branded as demonic (often erroneously by religious leaders) and working for the left-hand path in order to distort human evolution. This has included Lucifer, who is discussed further in the Venus book of this series – a planet with which he has a strong connection.

The Kabeira, also known as the Kabira, were ancient priest kings and related to the ancient Titans. They were giants in physical stature as well as of powerful intellect. In this way they could function as leaders for humanity and anchored the ray of will and power. They especially knew how to harness the power of fire and through this faculty were known as the Asuri. However karma was created through abuse of such powers, especially during Atlantis, when struggle ensued through attempting to dominate over sections of humanity. Such events led to many battles fought between the Kabira and the other leading factions, including the wizards and sorcerers. There was also a great war fought during Lemuria and Atlantis between some of the fallen angels and the gods remaining within the higher spiritual realm. Examples included the war between gigantic Titans and the ancient Greek pantheon of gods, led by Zeus.

The role of Mercury pertaining to the incarnation of gods, fallen angels and demons into the planet included the need to bring these higher spiritual beings into the correct time and space on Earth for their mission. Mercury awakened the subconscious memories that needed clearing within those humans receiving assistance from such higher beings. This enabled the new information to enter their physical nervous system and consciousness.

Through such integration humans are becoming more self responsible and consciously committed to their spiritual destiny on Earth. Consequently the spiritual realm can channel greater levels of alignment, knowledge and gifts to the human incumbent – freeing up the fallen gods and angels from their supportive role. In effect, Mercury helps to empower each human.

Overall character of the god

In summary, Mercury in myth is imbued with many qualities which at first sight appear to paint a contradictory character. These include:

- With sickle sword in hand he is ever ready to slay and aid those in battle on Earth.

- With his magic staff he is a conjurer of the spirits of the dead.

- He is a volatile and devouring aggressor for the mild mannered of humanity.

- He is the relentless and unyielding, yet seductive psychopomp as guide for dead souls, with a speed as quick as death.

- He is the spirit within gravestones and signposts.

- He rules over merchants, shepherds and cattle herders.

- He rules over thieves and deceivers and is the master thief.

- He governs deft guidance and sudden gains or windfalls. He is a master finder.

- He represents the divine innocence of the newborn, of becoming into the world.

- He interprets the spiritual meaning behind all material things.

- He is a god of procreation and fertility.

- The magical powers of plants are well known to him and he is a master alchemist-healer.

- He is the magical escort for travellers and all those on a journey.

- He is a transcendental guide and leader for humanity. He conveys the sum or total possibilities of all available pathways in life.

- He is variously shameless, gentle and merciful.

- He has a general divine readiness to help yet also a devilish joy at others' misfortune.

- He is masculine and audacious, yet also feminine and sensitive.

- He is both phallic and spiritual.

- He is a spirit or fellow of the night and enables the processes of forgetting, sleep, regeneration and dying.

Chapter 10

Mercury and the human personality

Mercury and forgetting

Forgetting is the opposite to the retention of an image, impression or thought within the mind. Humanity is plagued by a lack of memory, affecting many spheres of day-to-day thinking as well as deeper knowledge. However, this is ultimately of great benefit, with the influence of Mercury being particularly important.

It is the etheric body that imparts the ability to have memory and is affected by forgetting. The inherent nature of the etheric body is anabolic, propagating and building-up with repetitive-growth activity. In the plant kingdom it governs the growth of the typical species, with the upward growth of the stem and each leaf repeating the same basic shape as the last. The uppermost part of the stem transforms into a flower due to even higher (astral) subtle forces streaming towards the plant. Similarly etheric blueprints define the column of vertebral bodies in the human backbone, whereby each bone is more or less similar to the one below. The cranium or head is then shaped by blueprints from the astral, mental and spiritual bodies – as revealed by the air spaces within the skull and the greater differentiation of shape. These higher principles bring the repetitive etheric dynamic into final conclusion.

It could also be said that the plant is not open to truly individualised development during its life. The seed from which the plant derives effectively defines the whole future of the plant. However, in the human embryo, the genetic codes and fertilised germs cells from the parents do not fully define the whole of life development. This is due to the soul-spirit or ego forces that impart a sense of self and individual character, shaping the form and function of the developing being on many levels from physical to spiritual. Of course there may be within the child similarities and inherited features to its ancestors, but each human responds to this and to the environment in a peculiarly unique way. Alongside this lies the capacity for humans to receive education, a faculty beyond the plant. Whereas the plant responds to the Earth environment in a reactive manner, humans can co-create their environment and mould their destiny.

It is not the whole of the human etheric body that vitalises physical growth and the metabolism. There is a part of the etheric which is free to mobilise elsewhere, to vitalise the thinking life. This starts, in particular, from the age of around seven years. Before this the etheric body of the human baby and toddler is relatively firmly bound to its physical body, for which it provides growth forces. However the body of the child below the neck is especially fashioned from the genetic and germ cell (sperm and egg cells) blueprints of its ancestors as within the maternal womb. The head of the embryo additionally derives its blueprints from the past lives of the soul coming into this incarnation. Thus the newborn baby is really only present within its head and not even fully in that, hence the inability to control any body functions and to barely lift its head. The soul of the child eventually incorporates itself into the physical body to grasp it and claim it as its own. This process spans several (generally seven) years, culminating in the loss of its milk teeth (representing the ancestral blueprints) and emergence of its first set of proper adult teeth (see p.232).

Along the way it throws out of the physical and etheric bodies those parental/ancestral genetic and holding patterns it does not wish to retain, and this process manifests as febrile childhood infectious diseases. The fever is needed by the child to 'burn' out the obsolete ancestral information, which pours out as discharge. Suppression of fever by paracetamol or other analgesic drugs and dampening of the mucus by antibiotics leads to retention of such mucus, which becomes a culture medium for further microbial growth. This is because mucus is a gel-like substance, which becomes watery and runny when warm (hence pouring easily out of the body) but thick and sluggish when cooled (leading to glue ear, congested lungs, etc.).

If the incarnation of the soul proceeds normally to the age of seven years, the next seven-year cycle can properly begin. In this period, from the age of eight to fourteen, a freed part of the etheric body becomes loosened from its function of vitalising growth of the physical body. It then serves to energise the thinking, particularly along the lines of creative imagination, a faculty often noted by educators to open up in this period.

Although it is the astral body which receives sensory impressions (visual, auditory and so on), it is the function of the etheric body to hold these impressions so that they do not disappear. Perception occurs through the astral body, but memory through the etheric – which thus comes to hold all our memory pictures. Remembering is simply the ability to bring back to the astral body's awareness the stored memory picture within the etheric body.

Over the human life, the wealth of such memory stored within the etheric body provides for inward experiences that influence the individual's behaviour. There is an immense difference between the person who exercises a vital enthusiastic etheric body in order to learn during their life, to the lazy apathetic person whose etheric body is stagnant and in a rut. Effective learning and remembering depends on how much of the etheric body is mobile and free for storage (as opposed to simply providing vitality for physical body functions).

In truth, the etheric body never actually loses any of its stored memory pictures. Instead the lower personality forgets the vast majority of these etheric pictures, both short and long-term experiences. However the actual sense impression of, for example, something seen many years ago – such as a particular flower – is still within the etheric body as vivid as when first perceived.

There is a significant difference between a mental picture stored consciously within the memory and the same picture being forgotten at a later time. Upon being initially formed by sensory impressions from the external world, the mental image is enlivened and requires constant attention to maintain it. However this focus of attention causes consciousness to become diverted from attending to the present moment in time/space – through overly focusing on the image formation arising from an earlier time/space. When the image is forgotten, it not only remains present within the etheric body, but also can now work unhindered within the subconscious and superconscious realm. Only after this forgetting can the image be properly digested within the lower levels of consciousness in the etheric body and become of service to the human. It can then build up intelligence in the physical-etheric body that could not have formed if the image remained consciously and attentively in the head region. Without the ability to forget the etheric body would rapidly become clogged with memory images and the free mobile element of the etheric body would not be able to vitalise new creative impulses within the being. If the human received sensory impressions but was not able to release them, their consciousness would become overwhelmed by memory. Similarly insomnia can result through the inability to forget the many mental images acquired over the day. The ability to forget has therefore been a blessing to humanity over its evolution.

Forgetting also occurs between the soul's lives in earthly incarnations. After vacating a physical body, the soul undergoes an intricate process of review and reflection in the spiritual plane. It must plan out its future life in accordance with the karma needing balancing from its former incarnation. However, in order to properly incarnate into that next life, it must lay a veil of forgetfulness separating the awareness of the next personality from its former incarnations. Otherwise the personality of the next life would not be able to cope with the huge amount of data processing occurring at the soul-spirit level and within the astral body. Without forgetting there would be a thread of full awareness linking the earthly incarnations, which would hamper the ability of the personality of any one particular life from feeling free will and self-motivation. Without forgetfulness a human would not be able to develop or learn.

When there is too much conscious retention of memory-images within the etheric body, then those parts of the etheric body become hardened, stagnant, restricted and dried out. The liver, being the seat of the etheric body, is especially affected to create liver stagnation which can result in cirrhosis, becoming a hard and shrivelled organ relatively deadened to further impulses in life. The liver is regarded as the organ basis for the proper flow of emotional energy, in an abundant and enthusiastic manner. The heaviness and darkening of the liver energy is referred to as 'melancholy' or 'black bile'. The soul has bitter memories that impart a heavy weariness in the liver, making the etheric body feel unduly earthbound.

A brief survey of the processes after physical death is instructive: devachan is a name given to the spiritual realm the soul eventually enters after death of the physical body vehicle. However before this the soul must transit the astral plane, also known as kamaloka, because it cannot forget the desires, inclinations, hopes and belief systems of its former life. In this interim phase the soul must clear the mental and emotional memories it carries out of that earthly incarnation, otherwise it is not liberated enough to move onward. The soul departs from the physical body, which now falls into degeneration (no longer enlivened by the soul-spirit). Most of the etheric body is also left on Earth, gradually to decompose under the earthly laws of nature (notably sometimes etheric shells of energy become infused by discarnate entities to create poltergeist and ghostly phenomena, especially at sites of concentrated energy such as graveyards). During the first four days after physical death, the soul experiences a vast tableau of all the experiences within its etheric body, rather like a vivid flashback of its whole life. The soul does however take a small part of the etheric body away with it, called the etheric seed atom. This effectively carries a blueprint of the sum totality of experiences and memories within the former etheric body. The astral body carries the whole of the desires, sensory impressions, emotions and feelings over the incarnations of the soul. The astral body therefore must also review the impressions stored within it from the life just left. For this purpose the etheric seed atom vitalises the impressions streaming out of the astral body within the astral plane of kamaloka.

The soul can also peruse the akashic records (a library of the astral-based memories from all the lives of the soul). The etheric seed atoms retained from each individual life are used to vitalise the astral records.

However, for many souls, the etheric seed atoms have dense energy stuck in various realities within former lives. For example, the soul may have left its physical body with unrequited love interests, memories of broken hearts, unfinished tasks and various issues of unfulfillments. These cause an etheric seed atom to be tied to the Earth, often to relatives and loved ones left behind. The impressions from the astral body will thus also become trapped to such etheric ties to Earth and the soul may experience a long harrowing period of stagnation in the astral plane. Suffering within this realm occurs through the soul's inability to forget its connections with the physical earthly world, which stay hovering in front of it like a memory it cannot release. Indeed it may only become freed when relatives or colleagues release the soul from its unmet obligations on Earth, by themselves letting these go through acceptance and by detachment from their own bereaved suffering.

Through the facility of forgetting, the soul has the possibility to re-write the trials and tribulations it 'remembers' from its former lives on Earth, leading to a new form of liberation – one where it has actually stepped out of space and time limitations. The power of Mercury accelerates this process, which otherwise is a difficult and gradual effort of letting go. The transformation is represented by the waters of 'Lethe' and the river Styx, across which Mercury guides the dead souls to the next realm. This river imbues the soul with forgetfulness.

The next phase of devachan is within the higher spiritual planes beyond the astral plane. Here mental and spiritual qualities encompass awareness of the fifth, sixth and even higher dimensions of reality. The fifth-dimension concerns non-linear thought processing beyond space and time, and the sixth with collective soul awareness. Devachan is blissful to the soul; it is a period of rest and also for planning out the next possible incarnation, experienced with an enthusiastic anticipation. But the soul can only truly enter and experience devachan if it can adequately forget the memories brought up in the astral plane. The achievements of its former life can then be built into its next life in a truly creative way. Advanced human souls are able to completely empty the etheric seed atom and create an astral seed atom out of the digested astral body within kamaloka (in doing so these souls are being truly selfless without emotional attachments).

The moral of this section is that the soul should learn forgetfulness on an ongoing basis to avoid having to go through such a concentrated and often painful process after physical death. This is learning to surrender to the soul-spirit, to live in acceptance, peace and grace throughout one's life by constantly letting go of attachments, resentments, grudges, etc.

Stability of the personality

Mercury is involved in the development and stabilisation of the personality (lower ego), which is nonetheless an illusionary construct. It is a collection of self-imposed identities which the soul experiences in its present incarnation on Earth (Fig. 7-2). These include role models played in the various situations of life, belief systems, ambitions, hopes, desires, memories and learned behaviours from the external world. The personality is inherently unstable and any novel or transformative impulse could potentially destabilise its hold over reality. True reality is not that understood by the personality, the spiritual perspective of this material world being but maya or illusion.

Thinking

Viewing the outside world
A person may view the outside world to create mental images and thoughts, e.g. of a rose. The rose however has a life force, a soul, astral and etheric qualities, as well as aroma, taste, colour and shape. They are not really aware of how much of this totality has been grasped in the mental image.

Ownership of thoughts
When someone has a thought, it is fully endowed and permeated with all their spirit and mind. Everything within that thought is a part of the person, unlike the rose image, which is outside.

In truth a thought is most completely owned. Finding the relationship between self and thought, and between thought and the cosmos, provides awareness of the relationship between self and the cosmos. However, although they do not realise it themselves, most individuals do not have true thoughts. In their day to day life these are simply mental words, without spiritual substance or power. They are merely a flow of words, whether said out loud or retained internally. Hence the feeling inwardly of uncertainty as to what to believe or think. True thoughts are anchored to spiritual realities. Many people when they ask for an explanation on something are satisfied with an answer if it contains words with a familiar ring. This tendency often exists in intellectuals, philosophers, scientists and most people who call themselves 'thinkers'.

History of thinking
Modern intellectualised thinking started from the sixth to eighth century BCE. Before then, humanity experienced the world in pictures (this was the last phase of the old clairvoyance of the ancients). After this mental pictures evolved into logical analytical constructs. This especially began during ancient Greece, as illustrated by Socrates, Plato and Aristotle: this led to a denial or doubting of universal truths and concepts, causing a belief that these were merely words and names, without an actual basis in reality. This belief system, called 'nominalism', is widely held today. As an example we take the illustration of the cat; there is a cat in London, one in Paris, another in New York, etc. All of them are obviously separate cats. There does not appear to be a single universal cat linking them all together in the third-dimension. But in the upper dimensions, there exists a universal cat deva or spirit. The nominalist thinker would argue the concept of something universal, something that cannot be seen, is only an illusion. They would say that if there is a cat-in-general, then it should be perceptible. Because they cannot be shown this universal cat, they presuppose it must not exist.

Third-dimensional thinking
Because philosophers have considered thinking to be 'easy', blunders have been made within the belief systems of the world. In the realms of scientific theory and intellectual study, thoughts are imbued with

realism in order to create hypotheses and discover underlying truths behind material things.

For example in many economic theories a hundred *actual* pounds are not less and not more than a hundred *possible* pounds. It makes no difference if one thinks of a hundred as actual or possible in order to deduce a truth in the economy. Through such theories decisions are made for controlling the world economy. However in practical life, the difference between a hundred actual and a hundred possible pounds is exactly a hundred, which of course is a big difference. Imagine an individual needs a hundred pounds, they will obviously choose the hundred actual pounds over the hundred possible pounds. However when they do not need any money, then it could be argued that a hundred actual pounds is exactly the same as a hundred possible pounds.

The actual substance of thought and its true connection to words needs to be reclaimed. This has major significance to understanding the world, for humanity has reached such modes of thinking by no longer having soul experiences through their thoughts. People generally explain the world from their own perspectives and opinions. In terms of world history, historians explain the events of the twentieth century as stemming from causes in the latter part of the nineteenth century, and these were themselves caused by preceding events in the early nineteenth century, and so on for the earlier centuries. One speaks of cause and effect, a pragmatic history. In truth, other factors create historical events other than those that push from the past. Fresh influences always enter each period of time from the spiritual world and many events are created by human souls through their planning of earthly incarnations within the spiritual world.

Humans are not taught how to think properly and thus fall into misguided beliefs, following these blindly. Humanity chooses to believe the theories of scientists and philosophers. Yet a person would not choose to let their gas central heating be repaired by someone with no proper training in gas installations, and yet people follow the beliefs of others who themselves have not received the [spiritual] training in the realm of thinking. Instead humans must step out of these belief systems and cause their thoughts to move into the upper realms.

Multidimensional thinking

Third-dimensional thinking, no matter how philosophical, is hopeless for arriving at the universal truths. Upper dimensional thinking involves setting one's thoughts into movement through imagination. Nominalist thinking stops at an intellectual boundary line and does not contact group-soul and spiritual energy. To know the outer material world a person does not actually need thoughts but only a memory – to remember the form last seen, and carry this into their future experiences. This is a trap into linear space and time, depending on memory to get through life. However most individuals become concerned when losing their memory, believing they will no longer be able to cope. But these thoughts were merely words and real thinking requires an imaginative connection to the spiritual realm through meditation.

Transcendentalism (Mercury)

There is a mode of thinking associated with each solar system planet. Mercurian thinking is where the person feels there must be a spiritual reality beyond the outer external or material world. Furthermore this higher reality is not only behind all things, but also beyond their own personality and soul. Whereas the mystical thinker believes that spirit flows into their soul, the transcendentalist believes this must flow outside of their soul, and is therefore beyond their soul experience. The essence of something being transcendental ensures this reality stays beyond personal experience at all times.

The throat chakra

The personality is very much linked to the throat chakra, which provides a connection between the soul-spirit forces working through the head and the material etheric forces working through the body. At the level of the throat (and as part of the throat chakra) are the thyroid gland, parathyroid glands, brainstem, vagus nerve (part of), trachea airway

MERCURY AND THE HUMAN PERSONALITY

and the vocal cords. All these structures (Fig. 10-1) serve the flow into and out of the physical body of higher subtle bodies, the astral and spiritual bodies. The personality at this level can either facilitate or hinder the movement of spiritual currents into the body.

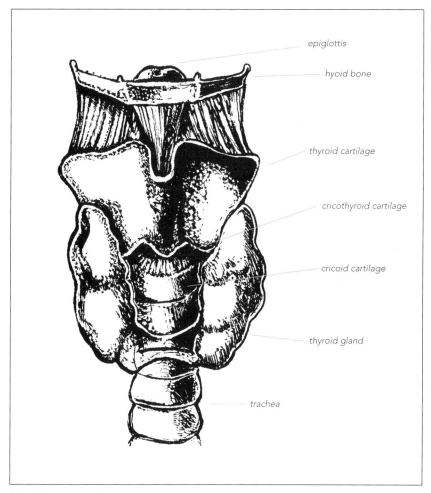

[Fig. 10.1] *Larynx (voicebox) anterior view. Speech is not simply vibration of the vocal cords under the influence of air currents but a faculty of soul-spirit, relying on movement of the astral body through the throat chakra. The astral body creates waves of compressed air within the region of the vocal cords, i.e. sound waves.*

Many humans, as yet asleep to their true spiritual nature, have blocks in these anatomical structures that limit the flow of spirit into the body. These can be described as implants, devices, matrices and veils. Implants in the brainstem block the conduction of spiritual thought energy into the spinal cord and peripheral nervous system, thus preventing the personality from acting on every thought and whim, until spiritual responsibility enables them to cleanse the brainstem. From that moment the soul has greater capacity to manifest their true ambitions on Earth. Similarly restriction in the larynx and vocal cords limits the true expression of spiritual power through the voice. Many esoteric and powerful energies of divine manifestation would thus only become apparent when the personality aligns to spirit and unblocks this region. Blocks at the upper airways and trachea lead to problems with breathing, such as chronic airways obstruction, chronic bronchitis, asthma and so on. These are typical diseases stemming from abuse of power in former lives, thus the soul experiences a limitation in its personal power in this life, even to the extent of not having enough power or energy to exert itself with ease.

Mercury is responsible for the proper, and hopefully graceful, unfoldment of the personality to merge with the soul-spiritual aspects of its being. Thus Mercury ensures the past life memories which require clearing are brought up one (or a few) at a time when the personality can both understand them in the present situational framework and also deal with them. It ensures that new information from the cosmos and spiritual realm streams into the personality at appropriate and relatively easy stages; otherwise the personality can feel overwhelmed by this new information and demands. Whenever the spiritual realm transmits a message to Earth, through the channel of Mercury, a crisis point of transformation is invariably induced. Too much and the world becomes too unstable a place (personalities would not have the time to complete their tasks before the next learning is brought about). This can be seen in Mercury as a planet, which had to slow down its rotational orbit to provide a proper basis for slowing down linear time on Earth. The spiritual beings working through Mercury are also closely involved with the shaping of time on Earth, and have been called the Spirits of the Ages and Spirits of Time.

If the foregoing is read in the light of the path of discipleship, it will be seen that along the journey the soul unfolds new faculties that alter the rulership of the planets over the various physical glands and chakras. In the spiritual disciple, Saturn comes to govern the throat chakra instead of Mercury. Concomitantly, the parathyroid glands activate and take over some of the essential functioning of this chakra. The parathyroid glands secrete parathormone, whose physiological role is to increase the level of ionised calcium in the blood. There are four tiny parathyroid glands, each smaller than a pea, lying behind the thyroid gland. Sometimes tumours occur in these glands, causing hyperparathyroidism, the symptoms of which include depression, constipation, lethargy and general malaise. Such a vague illness continues sometimes for years before medical doctors finally investigate these organs, to find abnormally raised levels of parathormone. If Saturn were activated prematurely (in terms of soul consciousness) in the average developed person then such an abnormal state can arise. Saturn would in such circumstances cause too deep a penetration by the personality structure into the mineral kingdom of Earth. The personality then feels too densely incarnated and too rigid in respect of life choices.

Conversely, Mercury allows the personality to function in a relatively scattered mode with respect to thoughts, actions and life choices. Reaching the stage of discipleship necessitates a Saturn activation, which provides the firmness of character to withstand the various trials and tribulations of the path, as well as solidifying the path. The disciple must now live in the present and not create illusion by projecting over-ambitiously into the future, nor stagnate the past by having rigid memory. The calcium vibration provided by the increased parathyroid activity provides the mineral substrate for manifesting the spiritual realm into the material world. Mercury then shifts to govern the brow chakra of the disciple, which undergoes a qualitative change in functioning. From now on, the brow chakra deepens the power of clairvoyance, thus the disciple learns to 'see' into distant realities – including far away stars and planets. Mercury provides the communicative and receptive quality required in this chakra for this purpose.

Chapter 11

Mercury within the human civilisation

Mercury in the Atlantean age

Many and profound were the uses of Mercury during this era of Earth's development. Atlantis was the supercontinent existing in what is now the Atlantic Ocean, although technically this is not absolutely accurate. It existed in a mixed second/fourth-dimensional realm rather than the current third-dimensional reality that humans consider to be the physical world. The second-dimension is somewhat akin to the subterranean and subconscious realm of the planet; it harbours elemental forces of nature and many demonic and angelic beings that assist humanity's evolution by guarding their subconscious and repressed emotions. Humans started to suppress their emotional memories into their subconscious, due to the lack of proper anchoring of the character forces of soul needed to deal with these.

It was especially important for the Atlanteans to suppress the unregulated sexual impulses inherited from the preceding age of Lemuria. Recall that during Lemuria there was the separation of the initially androgynous human species into the male and female types, starting the expression of heterosexuality and procreative reproduction. Formerly reproduction had been by budding and unisexual means, whereby a 'human' could create another being out of its own substance (the 'sweat-born'). Before sexual gender development the Lemurians had an open etheric link direct to the spiritual realm, and did not sense a separation between the material and spiritual. The division into the genders soon led to the fall, when these early Lemurians fell into the glamour and illusion of the material and sensory world. Their open crown chakra and related pineal gland began to descend into the brain substance and became sealed over in stages. The downfall of Lemuria led to its submergence under the sea floor, in the geographical region now represented by the Pacific Ocean.

The Atlanteans made extensive use of Mercury to suppress the Lemurian sexual impulses that still strove for uncontrolled expression, stemming from the sacral chakras of their physical bodies. The chakra that needed to develop within Atlantis was now the solar plexus, as a centre for the emotional life and development of astral powers. The need to raise the sexual energy stuck in their sacral to the solar plexus chakra became paramount. Mercury was well suited to suppressing the syphilitic miasm and sacral chakra of their initially mixed Lemurian/Atlantean bodies. Note that Mercury in organic form is still present in toxic amounts in many polluted rivers and oceans, and present within the tissues of sea-life such as fish. This reflects the early Lemurian beings, which were predominantly fish-like in body structure. The heightened and often frenzied sexual activity of fish (making huge numbers of fertilised eggs for their progeny) is a target for Mercury's toxicity. Note also how homoeopathic Mercury can be used to treat excessive and promiscuous sexuality, whether or not with precocious physical genital development. It suppresses the early activation of the sacral chakra in these children until proper emotional and soul development has occurred to thus enter the teenage life and activate sexuality in its proper place (see p.189).

Mercury was also used in Atlantis to develop their initially primitive lung structures. The lungs eventually became highly developed to harness the power of air and sound through their bodies. The Atlanteans used air in a manner reminiscent of modern air power tools, which are very powerful, clean and reliable. They could project air from their lungs and through their vocal cords so as to move objects, to fly, to sonically influence objects at a distance and even for sonic warfare. They developed shields to protect their own aura from sonic damage when attacked by others. Many souls who still have karma today from such past endeavours have health problems in their lungs, larynx, tonsils and in their speech. Example diseases are asthma, recurrent sore throats, tonsillitis and speech impediments.

During a stage in the development of their lungs, the Atlanteans resorted to 'polluting' the oceans with Mercury. This was not a deliberate act of environmental damage, but aimed toward developing lung structures containing alveolar air sacs within the initially sea-based creatures having predominantly gill lungs.

Later the Atlanteans used Mercury for the purposes of air transportation and communication systems. They had a sophisticated technology with respect to air travel, more advanced than humanity at present. They could harness the power of wind in powerfully subtle ways so as to alter the climate of the planet. Mercury as the air breathing metal was well suited to this task.

Much of the Mercury in use during Atlantis was the gaseous elemental form. In a future humanity, when Mercury will predominantly be in solid and also organic form at ambient temperature, there will be material levels of Mercury active in the human anatomy and physiology. Mercury will then assist the movement of information in and out of the human body. The future human body will function more clearly as a transmitting and receiving channel for spiritual beings to interact with those on the Earth material plane.

Mercury in ancient Egypt

In many of the mystery schools and ashrams of the ancient world Mercury was used as a powerful alchemical tool for working with consciousness. In Egypt, flasks of Mercury have been discovered in tombs dating from the second millennium BCE – gifts to the dead. Hermes, Thoth and Annubis are amongst the Gods entrusted with carrying the vibration of Mercury to the underworld, indeed they are each aspects of Mercury.

Of significance was the maintenance of reptile chambers (usually snake pits) under the major ashrams and mystery schools of initiation. The snakes provided the necessary subterranean anchor to receive and hold in place the cosmic and stellar vibrations channelled down to the site by the temple priests and spiritual masters. Snakes also hold the ancient curse within humanity of the fall; they carry the smear of losing the link to the spiritual realm through cultivation of the lesser ego. Of all animals, snakes represent cunning, deceit, slyness and manipulation. They often trigger fear and loathing in humans. This is not an accident, nor that the snake is represented as the precipitant for the fall in the story of Adam and Eve (by convincing humans to fall for sensory materialistic pleasures).

However, snakes are holding this guilt on behalf of humanity. When every human soul can re-align to their spirit and merge this with the fragmented lower ego or personality in an act of redemption and resurrection, then the snake will no longer need to store the blueprint of the fall. In the meantime snakes will continue to work energetically in the subconscious realm to maintain the enormous amount of suppressed and repressed debris within the collective subconsciousness of humanity. The role of Mercury is to carry those new cosmic frequencies needed by the subterranean snakes whenever the subconscious programs within humanity need adjusting. Part of this work requires the human soul, involved in a particular suppressed memory, to actually travel down to these depths and reclaim its missing soul fragments. This is another job for Mercury the psychopomp – to guide the human souls after their physical death to the underworld (see p.96).

One such initiation used by the ancient priests to prepare for this journey was to use mind-altering drugs (shamanic plants and substances, many of them now modern recreational drugs and used inappropriately for escapism). These would cause them to bypass their conscious mental body and slip their consciousness down into the subconsciousness. Their conscious mental body was much more immature than in most of present day humanity and the cerebral cortex (especially the frontal lobes of the brain) was only just starting to activate. An old form of mental functioning, from early Atlantean days, had been centred in the sympathetic nervous system, and based on emotional responses to the external world. The sympathetic nervous system was very suited to exploring the subconscious realm of consciousness – but it reacts to experiences therein by emotional states of fear, anxiety, courage etc., depending on the fortitude of the person. The ancient Egyptian initiations therefore involved the suppression of the conscious cerebral cortex-based mind, so as to regress into the sympathetic nervous system (which was more torso- and kidney-based) and thus activate immense emotional and elemental energies within themselves.

This technique is now obsolete and would be retrograde, causing harm to the present-day soul. The divine plan is now to raise the subconscious realm from the depths of the human psyche and the planetary matrix, and merge it with the more developed conscious mind. The waking consciousness and related cerebral cortex of the brain are now developed enough to cope with the heightened emotional surges that will be felt when the inner demons and shadows within the subconscious come to light. This will eventually free the snake species (group-soul of snakes) from carrying the burden of the fall. This process is represented by the raising of the kundalini serpent energy from the base of the spine to the head centres, to open the crown chakra and cause a flood of light to recycle down the body. Mercury assists the process of re-programming the physical body and lower chakras, enabling the ascension of energy to proceed safely.

Ancient gold and silver refining

Various ancient civilisations made extensive use of liquid elemental Mercury to extract and refine the small quantities of gold and silver within their respective ores. Much of this precious metal would be in fine distribution in the ore, but Mercury could dissolve and release it. This usage continued in the Romans who brought it from the Spanish mines. When the South American gold and silver mines became overworked and depleted, the Spaniards exported hundreds of tonnes of Mercury for extracting metal out of the poorer ores. Most of this Mercury came from Almaden in Spain.

There are spiritual causes behind every event in the material realm. Material events can therefore never be explained by other material events. There is a spiritual reason why Mercury was required to extract the gold and silver from the poorer ores. Metals, as also minerals and crystals, carry a vibration generated from the owner or person wearing it. Gold is a noble substance that in truth carries a refined message from the Sun of our solar system. It is a message of spiritual–material balance, courage, self-worth and unconditional love. It carries those attributes needed for a full and life-affirming opening of the heart chakra. However gold on Earth has for some time become polluted by the materialistic and greedy thoughts of humanity. It has become tainted by bloodshed and war in those who have fought over it, greed and pride in those who collect it, jealousy and envy in those who seek after it. These emotional vibrations stored in gold have distorted its true purpose on Earth. Such vibrations affect even that gold in ore as yet untouched by humanity, for all metal deposits of the same element resonate vibrationally with each other.

Since approximately the thirteenth century, a shift began in the evolution of human civilisation, to anchor a deeper awareness of the higher self and accelerate the path to mass ascension on Earth. This required a cleansing of gold on the planet, and Mercury was the best substance for this work. Through sublimation under Mercury, the gold received new blueprints from the spiritual and cosmic realm, bypassing those projected into it by humanity. This has paved the way toward a more unconditional and detached relationship between humanity and gold. The real purpose of gold mining on the planet has been for souls to realise the worth of the planet and of their material incarnations. Every time a human soul has mined, bought, owned or held gold during one of its incarnations, this lesson has been taught. In reality the personality can never possess that gold perpetually, for upon death of the physical body the soul leaves with its experiences, but not with the material things themselves. Thus for every possession of gold there will always be a letting go process, releasing the gold amulet or treasure back for use by the rest of humanity or Earth. Each experience with gold brings to the soul's awareness its own sense of personal abundance and self-worth. This is needed to clear the inner self-loathing and shame that had been programmed into the human psyche during the fall from grace (when humanity broke from the spiritual and divine realms to live out karmic and dualistic reincarnations on Earth).

Mercurial cleansing has lifted gold out of being an object of personal possession into an object of mass collective possession. In other words, the gold stored as federal reserve and in the vaults of the financial market technically belongs to the human race as a whole. This is not just a whimsical notion, for humanity is gradually learning to detach from the materialistic focus on gold and understand its true role to empower the inner forces of God will and power. Through gold the purpose of each human soul on Earth can be activated and facilitated. This is not a competitive lower egocentric design based on personal ambition and selfishness. To truly follow one's path requires gracefully being of service to assist others on their path. It is a state of collective soul consciousness, and anchors the sixth-dimension where the souls of all humans evolving through the Earth school can be contacted, reaching a truly democratic consensus on any decision that needs to be made by any individual soul.

The cleansing of silver from poor ores was required for a related purpose. Silver carries the energy of the Moon, which stores the memory of the personal and planetary past. It links the soul to the subconscious and the unconscious realms and by a process of reflective pondering regenerates such memories, bringing them up to surface consciousness for proper assimilation. However from the thirteenth century humanity needed to progressively break from its past. Humanity had developed along lines of tradition, religious subservience and a rigidified honouring of ancient wisdom. It was heresy to think in any other way than that dictated by tradition and the guardians of ancient knowledge (usually the priests). This thread linking humanity to the past was broken to bring about the change of consciousness needed for the age of reason and enlightenment. Science and logic now governed the thought processes of humanity; there was a denial of ancient wisdom, and a loss of faith or belief in reincarnation and other similar spiritual principles. This collective memory of the past was stored in the silver of the planet, which thus needed cleansing of such information.

Mercury not only cleansed, but provided a new faculty of the human soul with respect to the personal and planetary past memory. Through

Mercury's action on silver, it has now become possible to detach from the personal past and make it altogether objective. Souls can now travel into their past lives without feeling a subjective recapitulation of the past memory, enabling them to avoid feeling overwhelmed by the past memory as it surfaces. It has also allowed more advanced souls to travel into the past lives of others (as in therapists performing past life regression on their clients) and not become attached or personally affected by what comes up. This is now extending into the advanced soul's ability to re-write the past memory and history of the planet and human race with objective detachment. However, if done with subjective and personal agendas, such souls could re-write world history according to their personal desires and ambitions, which would be injurious to the collective. This helps explain the action of homoeopathic Mercury to stabilise the personality when too many past memories (whether from this or other incarnations) surface to overwhelm the consciousness or cause schizoid scattered states (see p.121). Silver, with the help of Mercury, will bring such memories up more clearly, without fearful distortion, and in a stable manner for the purpose of integration with the conscious mind. Note that silver is the metal of the Moon (see p. 52 for the astronomical relationship of Moon and Mercury).

Alchemical uses of Mercury

Although not strictly a material, the mercurial principle is related to Mercury. The three major principles are sal (or salt), sulphurous (sulphur) and mercurial. The salt principle represents the nerve-sensory dynamic, the activity of excretion and of deadened devitalised substance. Through it life is removed from an organism. The sulphur principle is enlivening, warming, vitalising and imbues substance with life and is the polar opposite of salt. The mercurial principle is the transformative dynamic quality that meets these two polarities and finds the point of balance, mediation and initiation. Through this last principle the ancient alchemists could make their secret and powerful mercurial water, by the finest arts of sublimation. Through this and other forms of Mercury, the alchemists extracted and purified gold and silver out of base metal. The real transformation was of course within their souls; the transformation of the lower self to the soul-spiritual self and the refinement of the physical body as a temple for the spirit.

Translated manuscripts from the Rosicrucian Order, dating from a convention of alchemists in 1777, reveal some of the secret lore pertaining to the Mercury principle. It is stated that the first matter of metals is a moist vapour, filled with the heat and fiery forces of the Earth and the Sun. This vapour is the Mercury principle, which is also called the heavenly water. It is liquid yet does not moisten. It can lead to all material things, whether in the mineral, plant or animal kingdom, through the influence of the sulphur principle. The sulphur principle leads to material manifestation of this heavenly water, providing the energetic receptacle for the warmth and life force to remain in place. This is further fixed into place by the salt principle. A finer distinction can be made between Mercury as the seed of metals, and quicksilver as the radical moisture of metals. The seed property of Mercury holds the germinal blueprint required for that metal to be able to transform into another form. The most perfect transformation possible for a metal is to change into gold. Imperfect transformation leads to crude substance, one of which is lead. The property of radical moisture on the other hand is the dynamic ability of Mercury to convey and carry that metal into the next stage of its transformative process.

An important work within alchemical lore, 'Currus Triumphalis Antimonii' (Triumphal Chariot of Antimony) by Basil Valentine, a German Benedictine monk, elucidates the properties of mineral Mercury thus:

'No animal or vegetable contains anything that can avail to fix Mercury; the attempt to do this has always ended in failure, because none of these substances have a metallic nature. Mercury is both inwardly and outwardly pure fire: therefore no fire can destroy it, no fire can change its essence; it flees from the fire, and resolves itself into an incombustible oil spiritually; but when it is once fixed, no cunning of man can volatilise it again. Then everything can by art be made of it that can be produced from gold, because after its coagulation it y resembles gold, seeing that it has grown from the same root, ng from exactly the same branch as that precious metal.'

Here is laid an alchemical secret of great spiritual significance, which explains why Mercury has retained its liquid nature over and above all the other metals. Mercury contains the blueprints for transformation of base metals into gold; thus the blueprint of gold is within the nature of Mercury. Homoeopathic Mercury similarly provides a subtle transformation within the body, preparing the way for the finer qualities of soul and spirit out of the base personality.

Further vital information can be gleaned from a passage in a rare volume of treatises, 'The Hermetic Museum', published in Frankfurt in 1678. In the volume titled 'The Open Entrance to the Closed Palace of the King' written by an anonymous sage (who may be Eirenaeus Philalethes), under a heading 'Of the Difficulty and Length of the First Operation':

'Some alchemists fancy that the work from beginning to end is a mere idle entertainment; but those who make it so will reap what they have sown – viz., nothing. We know that next to the Divine Blessing, and the discovery of the proper foundation, nothing is so important as unwearied industry and perseverance in this First Operation. It is no wonder, then, that so many students of this Art are reduced to beggary; they are afraid of work, and look upon our art as mere sport for their leisure moments. For no labour is more tedious than that which the preparatory part of our enterprise demands. Morienus earnestly entreats the King to consider this fact, and says that many Sages have complained of the tedium of our work. "To render a chaotic mass orderly", says the Poet, "is matter of much time and labour" – and the noble author of the Hermetical Arcanum describes it as a Herculean task. There are so many impurities clinging to our first substance, and a most powerful intermediate agent is required for the purpose of eliciting from our polluted menstruum the Royal Diadem. But when you have once prepared your Mercury, the most formidable part of your task is accomplished, and you may indulge in that rest which is sweeter than any work, as the Sage says.

There are those who think this Art was first discovered by Solomon, or rather imparted to him by Divine Revelation. But though there is no reason for doubting that so wise and profoundly learned a sovereign was acquainted with our Art, yet we happen to know that he was not the first to acquire the knowledge. It was possessed by Hermes, the Egyptian, and some other Sages before him; and we may suppose that they first sought a simple exaltation of imperfect metals into regal perfection, and that it was at first their endeavour to develop Mercury, which is most like to gold in its weight and properties, into perfect gold. This, however, no degree of ingenuity could effect by any fire, and the truth gradually broke on their minds that an internal heat was required as well as an external one. So they rejected aqua fortis and all corrosive solvents, after long experiments with the same – also all salts, except that kind which is the first substance of all salts, which dissolves all metals and coagulates Mercury, but not without violence, whence that kind of agent is again separated entire, both in weight and virtue, from the things it applies to. They saw that the digestion of Mercury was prevented by certain aqueous crudities and earthly dross; and that the radical nature of these impurities rendered their elimination impossible, except by the complete inversion of the whole compound. They knew that Mercury would become fixed if it could be freed from their defiling presence – as it contains fermenting sulphur, which is only hindered by these impurities from coagulating the whole mercurial body. At length they discovered that Mercury, in the bowels of the earth, was intended to become a metal, and that the process of development was only stopped by the impurities with which it had become tainted. They found that that which should be active in Mercury was passive; and that its infirmity could not be remedied by any means, except the introduction of some kindred principle from without. Such a principle they discovered in metallic sulphur, which stirred up the passive sulphur in Mercury, and by allying itself with it, expelled the aforesaid impurities. But in seeking to accomplish this practically, they were met with another great difficulty. In order that this sulphur might be effectual in purifying the Mercury, it was indispensable that it should itself be pure.'

Ancient and modern therapeutic uses of Mercury

Mercury is one of the oldest of all medicines and was used in ancient Egypt, Assyria and Babylonia. One formulation was a mixture in grease as an ointment. It became increasingly used as a general medicinal from the mediaeval ages till the twentieth century. Thus it was the main therapeutic agent for treatment of syphilis and leprosy, especially the former after widespread prevalence of this disease from the sixteenth century.

Various treatment regimens developed, the main ones being inunction and fumigation. Oral ingestion was rarely used. Inunction involved the rubbing of mercurial ointment into the skin. Fumigation involved the patient being well greased and then sitting on a heated tray containing Mercury sulphide or other such compound. The Mercury vapour thus absorbed into their skin through the grease. Doses were titrated until the onset of salivation (drooling), sweating and gum inflammation. Little did many of the physicians realise these were actually toxic effects of Mercury and many patients met worse deaths than from the original disease itself. It was however used as a general medicinal for all sorts of ills, again often ending the patient's life through the toxicity. The use of Mercury provided the name 'quacks', for quacksalver referred to a prescriber of quicksilver. Even up to 1929 pharmaceutical compendiums often contained more than a hundred mercurial preparations – as gargles, eyedrops, soaps, ointments and oral pills.

Pink disease

This disease, also called acrodynia, was caused by the use of Mercurius chloride in teething powders and skin ointments, especially on children. It was common during the early part of the twentieth century, and almost disappeared when such teething powders were removed from the market in 1954. The symptoms displayed by the baby or child was constant crying, extreme photosensitivity, putrid discharges from the body, loss of appetite, flaccid muscle tone, teeth decay and excessive teeth grinding, lung failure, excessive sweating, arthritis and muscle pains, poor co-ordination, poor concentration, loss of confidence and shyness. All these symptoms of Mercury toxicity can be found in the homoeopathic picture of Mercury in the materia medica (see p.7), whether in children or adults.

Autism

This is a disease of early childhood with the following features:

- Abnormal social interaction when relating to others, showing extreme aloneness, lack of attachment, failure to cuddle or touch and avoidance of eye contact.

- Language impairment with a lack of understanding

- Ritualistic and obsessive/compulsive behaviour with insisting on the same, resisting change, rituals and habits, excessive attachment to certain objects and repetitive acts.

- Delayed or uneven intellectual development.

The diagnosis is only made after the age of thirty-six months. Many of the features of autism match those of Mercury poisoning, and have been attributed to the thimerosal within many vaccinations. This compound is 50% ethylmercury and is used as a preservative in the preparation. It was introduced into vaccines from the 1930s and coincided with the first significant reports of autistic children. A link between the two seems plausible considering the massive increase in vaccination alongside the increasing incidence of autism.

Common features of Mercury poisoning and autism thus include the following:

- Extreme under-confidence with shyness, social withdrawal and introverted states. A lack of direct eye contact and avoiding conversation.

- Mood lability with low mood switching to gaiety without any external context. Also a dull apathetic facial expression, with staring absently.

- Mental retardation and poor memory.
- Self-harm, including banging one's head.
- Anxiety, restlessness, nervousness and panic attacks.
- Speech deficit, poor comprehension of other's conversation, or abnormal sensitivity to sound and noise.
- Insomnia or difficulty falling asleep.
- Aversion to touch.
- Poor co-ordination, clumsiness and walking on their toes.
- Abnormal tremors, jerking movements and twitches of muscles.
- Photophobia.
- Excessive sweating.
- Anorexia or loss of appetite.
- A tendency to masturbate.

An even worse effect has been caused by certain influenza vaccines that contain both Mercury and aluminium, and after several annual inoculations of these the toxic accumulation of both metals can cause severe states of dementia.

Amalgam fillings in dentistry
Modern amalgams tend to contain mostly Mercury with a silver alloy and some tin and copper. They are designed to withstand the high mechanical pressures of biting and chewing and also the range of temperatures experienced through very hot and cold drinks. Various symptoms, such as headaches, behavioural changes and other features fit with Mercury toxicity. As well as the constant chemical leaching of

Mercury into the body from the amalgam, there is arguably an electrical effect from current passing between amalgam deposits through the alkaline saliva within the mouth. This electrical current swamps the much smaller current coursing through the nearby central nervous system. Disorders that can thus arise include chronic tension of the temperomandibular joint, facial paralysis (e.g. Bell's palsy), migraine headaches, visual and hearing defects, multiple sclerosis, epilepsy, cerebellar and spinal degeneration, dementia and Parkinson's disease amongst many others.

Syphilis, AIDs and HIV
From the spiritual perspective the illness of syphilis has now penetrated deep into the human species. It is present within the human gene pool and at a miasmatic level it has run for innumerable generations. It is deeply embedded within the past life records of human souls. It would take more than a short course of homoeopathic Mercury to rid this ailment, and it is still rampant in its many guises today, such as multiple sclerosis, AIDs and HIV infection, dementia of all kinds and most forms of heart disease. Many human souls over their last few incarnations have had to experience physical body demise with some form of toxic medicine in their system. This toxicity continues to act on the etheric shell left over after the soul vacates the physical body. The effect of Mercury has thus continued long after its initial administration. It is preparing the way for a new cycle of creativity, including sexual. Humanity has passed through a mercurial stage over the latter part of the twentieth century whereby human souls anchored the vibration of Mercury into their sacral chakras. The clearing of obsolete blueprints from the egg and sperm cells produced by the gonads has enabled many humans to form a new kind of sex cell – one that can receive new and divine blueprints.

Overcoming toxicity in the chakras
This facilitates the coming of a Venusian age as pertains the sacral chakra, and many of the future incarnating souls will have a strong sense of refinement, creativity, harmony and artistic talent to a level never before attained on Earth. Already many of the babies incarnating at the

current time are very advanced and wise souls. Despite limitations in the etheric and subtle bodies of their parents, these babies are coming in with almost full self-realisation of their innate mastery and Christ-consciousness. This is a Venus impulse, and has been prepared by the toxic effects of Mercury on the sacral chakras, limiting excessive Lemurian karma from penetrating into modern humanity.

Mercury and Mad Hatter disease

Mercury poisoning was a well-known occupational hazard of hatmaking, where Mercuric nitrate was used to convert animal fur into felt. An important centre of hatmaking, in Danbury, Connecticut, USA led to the disease being called the 'Danbury shakes'. An illustration is also provided by the character Mad Hatter in 'Alice in Wonderland'. Patients suffered personality changes, tremor and shakes, depression, fatigue, anxiety and fears. Other features included blushing easily in social settings, excessive shyness, paranoia about being watched, avoiding people, aggressive tendencies, agitation and a desire to return home.

Production of mirrors with Mercury and tin

Many mirrors made from the middle ages until the early part of the twentieth century were made with an amalgam coating of Mercury and tin on glass. An occupational hazard of the mirror makers was their early demise from Mercury poisoning. However the spiritual consequence of the use of such mirrors was the activation of the solar plexus chakra within humanity. Tin is the metal of Jupiter and relates to the functioning of the liver, which is the seat of tin forces. Tin and Jupiter also represent the king of the ancient gods, of superior rank to Mercury who is his messenger.

For most of humanity until only a few hundred years ago, the solar plexus chakra was very closed, and influenced greatly by residual Atlantean karma. This was the karma of emotional control, domination, power struggles and manipulation of others even at a distance. The key karmic activity in Atlantis was theft and suppression in all its various forms, including theft of soul parts or fragments of energy and consciousness from others. These patterns had perpetuated the feudal caste systems of land ownership, whereby most of humanity was subservient to landlords esteemed above them in position. A human could work hard all his life, and yet die destitute and still owing his/her landlord a huge sum, of course payable through any of his family left behind (even to the extent of enslaving his children). Most of humanity could not mount enough emotional power within their solar plexus centres to overcome the sense of frustration and anger into a positive zealous energy of revolution and self-determination.

This situation had of course changed by the time of reformation such as the French Revolution. The use of Mercury–tin mirrors actually reflected back to the observer the suppressed Atlantean energy within their solar plexus chakra. This was an unconscious experience for most souls in that the solar plexus and liver have a poor nervous system compared to a rich metabolic activity. Humanity is not supposed to be too conscious of the activity within the solar plexus chakra, otherwise much nervous energy would be wasted in consciously balancing the digestive and metabolic realm instead of simply letting the physical and etheric body get on with it. Through the surfacing of old Atlantean memories, filtering from their subconscious minds into their present incarnation, humans began to increase their sense of emotional self, to the point of emotional empowerment and development of a stronger character.

Contemporary medical and scientific ages of Mercury

In the present timeframe, Mercury has become a tool for the modern medical physician. It is used for temperature measurement, where it's quick expansion and contraction under ambient heat and cold provides a sensitive gauge. This is reflected in the intense heat the planet Mercury faces toward the Sun, yet with freezing cold temperatures on the side facing away. Similarly, in the homoeopathic picture of Mercury, the patient is immensely sensitive to the effects of heating or cooling, with aggravation of symptoms in each direction. Mercury is used in blood pressure monitors and until the recent past: as a medical disinfectant, as ointments for treating many skin diseases, syphilitic ulcers and eye diseases of all kinds. These were of course banned when the toxic effects were realised. It is still however used as an amalgam in dentistry, despite the increasing evidence of its chemical and electrical toxicity from within the mouth.

These toxic effects of Mercury are being compounded by the increased amount of other forms of Mercury passing through physical bodies today. Thus much toxicity from Mercury has resulted from its use within many allopathic vaccinations, where it is used in organic form as a bacteriostatic to limit the pathogenicity of the microbe. It is exceedingly artificial and foreign to the human immune system, which reacts to this contaminant with a hyper-stimulated production of antibodies. However many of the large numbers of antibodies produced become auto-immunogenic, attacking parts of the person's own anatomy, causing such increasingly common diseases as rheumatoid arthritis, diabetes, hypothyroidism, multiple sclerosis and many others.

Another modern form of Mercury toxicity is the vibration within telecommunication, mobile phone and satellite systems. These actually use the vibration of Mercury to guide the signal, even though humanity does not yet realise the spiritual dimensions of this technology. The problem is that many physical bodies are simply not healthy and robust enough to handle the rarefied and multidimensional energetic signals beaming into their nervous systems almost constantly during modern life. Information technology and the speed of communication has led to an immense activation of the nervous system, speeding up the action potential along nerve axons and increasing synaptic junction activity between cells. This is depleting the nervous system of vital chemical neurotransmitters, causing such diseases as Parkinson's disease and depression, and generally wearing down the nerve-sensory system. Chronic fatigue syndrome, stress and depression are the results.

Homoeopathic Mercury is a vital remedy for clearing the effects of such excessive vibrational pollution of the human body. This period of increased toxicity of Mercury within the nervous system is however preparing the way for a future development of the nervous system, when humanity will have a much more active brain and spinal cord than presently. Science already acknowledges that less than 10% of the brain is used by a 'normal' human. In the future, humanity will have activated latent energetic centres within the nervous system. There will be etheric changes, such as upward extension of the brain (reminiscent of the high domed heads of certain Egyptian head-dresses and gods), and have a double spinal cord. The pituitary, hypothalamic and pineal glands will all enlarge to cope with the increased reception of divine spiritual energy. The cerebrospinal fluid will be faster flowing to provide a route for the higher subtle thought vibrations as well as for channelling activity.

Elemental and inorganic Mercury compounds are used in the manufacture of scientific instruments (such as thermometers and barometers) and electrical equipment (such as switches, oscillators, batteries, electrodes, meters, mercury vapour lamps, X-ray tubes and solders). Recent past uses of Mercury included the plating, tanning, dyeing, photographic, pharmaceutical and artificial silk industries. Organic Mercury compounds have been used to make disinfectants, fungicides (such as in paint and for treating seeds), antiseptics, herbicides, preservatives and for denaturing alcohol.

A major source for environmental contamination has been through the mercurial fungicide treatment of seeds. Studies have found over 1200 microbes in or on many seed types. Killing these is considered of value to improve the chances of germination and limit crop disease. However such fungicides have poisoned whole human communities, as well as contaminating the soil, surface and ground water for many years to come. It is interesting to note that esoterically Saturn rules seeds, and the planet Mercury is responsible for releasing the correct saturnine codes out of the ancient past (on an as needed basis) for present day humanity to deal with.

The modern scientific laboratory uses copious amounts of Mercury, in the various switches, measuring instruments and pumps, both for its electrical and chemical properties. Mercury is also used to extract air from matter and the atmosphere and for the production of artificial vacuums. The ancients knew of the power of the vacuum, but it had a negative connotation for them and was called 'horor vacuui' (the horror of the vacuum). A vacuum was abhorrent to the ancients for it represented the de-creation of matter, and was the reverse of the divine infusion of God's energy into matter. God imbued life into the clay, dust and mud of Earth to form living beings such as human. By removing air from living substance, humanity goes in the reverse direction of God. This is the direction of anti-matter and actually attracts demonic and ahrimanic (satanic) entities into the vacuum. Nothing is ever actually completely empty, but becomes filled with the energy and consciousness of beings which humanity are as yet unable to measure.

The extensive use of Mercury within science and through experimentation has however resulted in an unexpected outcome for scientists. Metallic Mercury within their instrumentation is already sensitive to the movement of the planets within the solar system, through its resonance with planetary Mercury. However the use of vacuums and other controlled environments (such as de-fuming cupboards) within many scientific experiments actually sensitises the Mercury metal to a far-flung cosmic influence. The starry heavens have been brought into the scientific experiment. Of course scientists have not taken into consideration the effect the movement of solar system planets (or indeed the stars within the galaxy, universe and cosmos) have on the outcome of their experiments. It is however a major cause for experiment failure, unexpected results and the lack of reproducibility. The ancients knew of the influence of the macrocosm (heavenly, cosmic and spiritual realms) on earthly activities. The alchemists of old would advise casting an astrological chart to assist the timing for certain herbal and mineral manufacturing processes. It is an irony for science that the aspect of Mercury particularly working through their experiments is the confidence trickster and inconstant liar. Thus much of their work comes to nought but adds to a mountain of illusionary data trying to explain the material realm from the perspective of mechanical forces.

Chapter 12

Mercury in the biological and cellular realm

The relationship between cells and the whole organism

Complex multi-cellular organisms with internal organs use the vibration of Mercury to harmonise the lines of communication between the individual cell and the whole. Modern biology attempts to understand the functioning of the whole from an understanding of the cellular part. This is, however, impossible, for the cell cannot contain the divine intelligence of the soul-spiritual self, from which stems the sense of character and I-ness that guides the physiology of the organism. The soul-spirit in fact imparts to the individual cell the sense of freedom and individuality within this whole, but on condition that the cell functions in harmony with the whole. The cells make a promise to be of service and not injurious to the organism, in exchange for a certain sense of self-determination.

This individuality of the cells becomes apparent when the cell is isolated from the rest of the organism, as in cell cultures within the laboratory, in blood tests, pathology specimens and so on. That a cell can have an independent life when provided with appropriate nutrient media and stable conditions has given modern science the notion that the cell does not need the whole organism in a strict sense for its proper sense of place. Material science also presumes that the whole organism could be understood from mere conjunction of the activities of all the individual cells. There is the notion that the intelligence defining the activities of the organism, from the most mundane (such as digesting food) to the sublime (such as appreciation of art), is simply a consequence of the chemical and electrical activity of certain cells (in the gastrointestinal and brain respectively).

The removal of cells from the body, however, leads to a subtle but profound distortion of the fine field of energy supervising the whole body. This field of energy, variously called prana, chi, etheric energy, morphogenetic field, carries a blueprint originating from the divine spiritual realm and transmitted to the physical body. Without this etheric field the physical body would collapse like a heap of dust. The etheric contains the scaffolding for holding the physical body and the information matrix that guides the chemical reactions within the metabolism. These metabolic chemical reactions are not simply random processes, but are led by an intelligent consciousness, the soul-spirit, which stamps its imprint throughout the etheric body.

Diseases due to cellular separation

When a cell falls astray from collective control, the consequences include various pathologies such as allergy, autoimmune attack of the body, cancer formation and chronic mucus production. Allergy arises from the abnormal perception of self and the environment, partly from a loss of self-identity within the cells and the immune system, and partly from a rift in the defence chi (wei chi in Chinese medical terminology, a subtle layer of energy at the auric margin and skin). Thus the immune system mounts a hypersensitive defence against a foreign agent. Autoimmune disease results from the abnormal antibodies produced as a reaction to a distorted internal body image with respect to the environment. The protein antibodies attack the 'normal' tissues of the physical body, causing tissue destruction through chaotic inflammation. This is a modern version of the syphilitic trait, i.e. self-destruction of tissue.

Cancer results from the abnormal cells living a life independent of the blueprints streaming from the higher subtle bodies under the guidance of the soul-spirit. The etheric body at the region of the cancer has separated in a schizoid manner from the astral (emotional), mental and spiritual (awareness) bodies. This part of the etheric thus no longer holds the correct blueprints for control over the physical cells in that region, which consequently live under their own laws. Invariably the cancer is composed of undifferentiated cells with their own blood supply, due to the lack of higher guidance properly differentiating the cells.

Chronic mucus results from the hyper-stimulated B lymphocyte and general white cell activation, leading to large numbers of such cells dying as they over-produce antibodies or consume debris and allergens. Dead white cells mixed with water form pus or mucus. In a sense this process represents the decay of obsolete and ancient information stored in the etheric and physical body. Recall that Mercury works in conjunction with Saturn to unearth ancient knowledge within the human psyche and body, for example incomplete past lives and sclerotic ancestral memories. Before such old baggage consumes a soul the etheric body is invited to release it as mucus. The white cell is the basic cell type used for storage of old patterns based on duality, survival positioning and material separation from spirit. Thus it is suited for overcoming foreign entities and defending the body of the self from external harm. However in large part the white cells have become dinosaurs, causing more harm to the body than good, through their excessive reactions to microbes, allergens and toxic chemicals. It is the response of the immune system that causes the symptoms of infection and inflammation, such as fever, pus discharge, pain and swelling. Without an immune reaction there would be no symptoms.

This does not imply that a microbe would otherwise go on to engulf the immunologically apathetic organism. Rather the reverse, for foreign entities such as microbes would live in symbiotic harmony with the organism. The human immune system is currently undergoing a massive re-programming to clear away the duality-based survival codes of the past. This is necessary to enable the next level of functioning of the immune system, which is to provide a crystalline communication system between the cosmos/environment and the soul/body. The immune system will then learn from that which is foreign and not-self, rather than attacking this in a act of fearfully defending the integrity of the body. Analogously the blueprint of human consciousness is changing from duality to unity. Duality is a belief that external objects and events cause internal feeling. Unity is knowledge of the true higher and inner plane of reality as the cause for subjective states, that the external world is a reflection of this inner state of being.

Mercury is the key vibration to prepare these changes in the immune system and etheric energy field. Thus homoeopathic Mercury treats the above four diseases as caused by the fragmentation of the subtle bodies from the physical-etheric. It deals with chronic allergies, cancers, autoimmune destruction and mucus congestion. Mercury tends to bring all detached cellular and other processes back into the fold of the organism. It treats any separatism within the organism. This property is also revealed in metallic Mercury's ability to scatter into multiple droplets upon falling onto a surface, and yet to rapidly reconstitute into a single drop. It contains the forces required to form the multicellular organism as well as the governing unicellular whole being. Mercury also contains the forces of death and life needed to respectively restrain and enliven cells within the organism. If there were only life forces at work, without catabolism, breakdown or destruction of tissue, then a tumour process would readily occur. Death of cells enables recycling of the old and infusion of a new blueprint for cellular guidance. When Mercury's death forces are blocked from proper expression in the body physiology, then syphilitic auto-destructive processes again take their hold (where the catabolic breakdown dynamic within the metabolism has cramped inappropriately into the wrong direction).

Influence on digestion

Another key influence of Mercury is within the process of digestion and assimilation of food. Within the gastrointestinal tract the food is broken down into basic constituent particles. The large polymerised organic molecules such as proteins and carbohydrates are catabolised (broken down) to small organic molecules just short of the point of becoming mineral (i.e. not all the way to the atomic elemental level). Thus proteins are degraded to amino acids, carbohydrates to simple sugars and fats to fatty acids and cholesterol. The simpler constituents are then absorbed and travel in minute droplet form predominantly to the liver, through the portal vein. The droplet form reveals an essential function of Mercury here. The liver is the seat of the etheric body and the centre of the physical body's metabolic life. It has strong anabolic or building up properties, which is the dynamic of the etheric. By this means the liver can build up the particulate assimilated food substances to each other, forming complex polymer molecules again – only this time imbued with the character of self. The liver has the warmth energy of the soul-spirit flowing into it, which provides the necessary blueprints the liver requires, defining the proteins, fats, carbohydrates and other polymers with the right morphology.

Mercury is active at several points within this whole process. Firstly it prevents the broken-down constituents of food within the gut lumen from living an independent life of their own. It prevents activities which would otherwise arise such as bacterial fermentation and overgrowth, or flatulent gaseous build-up from the catalytic enzyme activity. Once the particles are absorbed into the blood stream, Mercury facilitates the etheric body in its function of enlivening this stream, preventing the broken down particles from stagnating in the portal blood or undergoing mineral deposition. Mercury also mediates the blueprints from the soul-spirit into the etheric body, thus providing the proper internal environment for anabolic creation of body substance, centred in the liver. If the blueprints from the soul-spirit are poorly infused, then food particles stream past the liver into the general systemic circulation. Also the improperly broken down foodstuff leads to fragments of basic constituents still bound to each other upon absorption through the gut wall. Thus remain, for example, short chain fragments of amino acids or chains of sugar molecules not fully broken down to single sugar molecules from the main carbohydrate polymer. These fragments retain the etheric blueprint of the former plant or animal from which they came, and through this maintain an energetic link to the group-soul of that species. The eventual result is a food allergy, whereby the rest of the human body and its immune system must react to the fragments bypassing the gastrointestinal system. It also points to a karmic relationship between the human soul and the particular nature group-soul working through the food, stemming from a past life which again has remained unresolved.

On the other hand, Mercury may act inappropriately and excessively to guide the blueprints and soul-spirit consciousness too deeply into the physical and etheric body. Mercury did after all represent the psychopomp, guiding souls into the underworld after physical death. This, in the context of the biological sphere, leads to an intense catabolic breakdown of the foodstuffs to produce mineralised products of digestion. This is alien to normal digestion, for the end products of food breakdown in the gut lumen must still be living organic molecules, albeit much smaller than their previous polymer form. Broken down to elemental forms, such carbonaceous decay products, ammoniums, sulphurous minerals etc. are absorbed through the gut wall, causing widespread deposition within the body. Diseases which can manifest include stones (renal, gallbladder), arthritis, sclerosis within blood vessels (such as ischaemic heart disease, thrombosis of arteries and so on) and excessive connective tissue hardening diseases (such as lupus or scleroderma). These are all syphilitic diseases, again revealing the essential relationship between Mercury imbalances and syphilis.

Mercury and syphilis

The nature of bacteria and the spirochetes
Micro-organisms are part of the normal cellular community within nature. Thousands of such cells perform valuable functions within the soil, atmosphere and water cycles of the planet. Very small numbers mutate into pathogenic strains and become labelled as specific types of bacteria, virus, parasite or protozoa etc. Of these, generally, bacteria represent obsolete information within the etheric body that ultimately becomes shed as mucus (this containing the past cellular information in the form of dead white cells).

Specific bacteria can appear upon particular disorders in the metabolism of metals, minerals and organic molecules within the human body. The family of bacteria linked most to mercurial metabolic processes is the spirochete group. These are typically long and slender in shape, tightly coiled and able to move within their medium. Their natural environment is aquatic and within some animal populations. Whereas most are benign, some cause disease in humans such as syphilis, an infectious disease due to the species Treponema pallidum. This is predominantly a disease of humanity. It affects many systems of the body and can last for several decades with a long period of latency or dormancy. It can be transmitted congenitally to the newborn. The immune system, in responding to the bacteria, can cause even more tissue destruction than the bacteria itself.

Homoeopathic miasms
To understand the syphilitic miasm it is important to understand the spiritual principles behind the concept of miasms. A miasm is an inheritance or predisposition to a particular mode of disease. It is the peculiar constellation of symptoms and signs that a person displays in reaction to a disease trigger that defines a particular miasm. It is based on parental and ancestral patterns of disease which have been passed onto the person through the genetic code (which is not itself the chromosomes but the morphogenetic field of information that the genetic code relays to the physical body). It is also based on the person's personal biography of disease, stemming from their past lives and from experiences in the current incarnation (see p.86).

There are three main miasms in homoeopathic philosophy and effectively the other miasms (tubercular, cancer, radiation, heavy metal, petrochemical, drug, vaccination and so on) are variants of the basic three. These are psora, sycosis and syphilis. It is beyond the scope of this book to discuss these in depth, but the keynotes will be outlined. The basic spiritual causation behind all miasms is the formation of disease as a result of separation from the spiritual realm. It is a result of the fall of humanity. The lower bodies (physical, etheric, emotional and lower mental) thus feel out of synchronicity and out of harmony with the upper bodies (astral, higher mental and spiritual bodies). The lower personality during an incarnation feels separate from the true source of its energy, i.e. the spirit. The specific reaction of the soul to the separation of the personality is displayed by the particular miasm.

The key feature of psora is underactivity and low resistance to illness. Patients are apathetic, listless with multi-organ weakness, yet with a tremendous itching of the skin. The nuance of the separation story displayed by psora is the feeling within the soul of apathetic depression and lack of desire to experience the path ahead on the material realm. The soul therefore tries to overcome this sluggish tendency by stimulating the cleansing forces of sulphur in an attempt to detoxify the burdened lower bodies of the incarnation.

The sycotic miasm is characterised by overgrowth, excessive mucus production and tumour formation. The separation story manifest here is the soul excessively compensating for its lost connection with spirit by doing too much on the material plane, but often thereby incurring karma for itself.

The syphilitic miasm is characterised by destructive activity, often with ulcer formation and necrosis of tissues. The soul compensates for separation by attempting to align the higher with the lower bodies but in a distorted and fragmented manner. Thus signals from the spiritual realm are not received clearly, leading to cramp of the tissues from the jamming of the spiritual signals. This pattern of distortion of the higher blueprints with consequent tissue destruction is prevalent throughout the clinical features of syphilis.

General morphology and motility of spirochete bacteria
Spirochete bacteria (one type being the cause of syphilis) are composed of an internal semi-rigid cell wall and an outer flexible cell sheath. This internal wall effectively forms what is known as a protoplasmic cylinder with a layer of periplasmic substance between this and the outer sheath (Fig. 12-1). Motility is due to many flagella that are connected to each pole. However, unlike most other bacteria, the flagella do not flex or move outside of the cell boundary but remain within the periplasm. They are thus known as endoflagella. Since they tend to extend for two-thirds the length of the cell there is overlap with the endoflagella from the opposite pole about the middle of the bacteria.

HOMOEOPATHY OF THE SOLAR SYSTEM: MERCURY

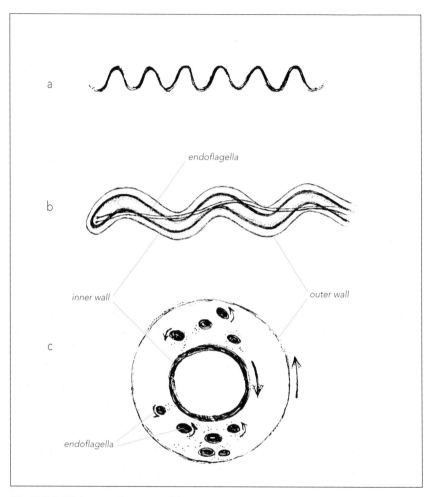

[Fig. 12.1] Syphilis bacterium, Treponema pallidum: (a) microscopic, (b) expanded microscopic, (c) transverse section showing position of endoflagella. Note the endoflagella between the inner wall or protoplasmic cylinder and the outer wall. The directions of rotation of each wall and the endoflagella are indicated.

The endoflagella rigidly rotate or spin (rather than contracting and swinging) and through resonance cause rotation in the outer flexible sheath in the same direction. However the inner partially rigid cell wall is made to rotate in the reverse direction through torsion effects. This creates a force on the protoplasmic cylinder, causing it to flex. Thus, despite not extending beyond the cell border, the endoflagella rotation leads to a spinning type irregular motion of the whole bacteria. This is rather like a corkscrew movement, rotating and spinning about the central body axis.

However, one cannot explain the motility of cells and organisms simply through mechanical forces. It is the astral body under the guidance of the ego or self-consciousness that leads to motion of the physical vehicle of the organism. Spirochetes and Treponema pallidum bacteria are the result of a disordered Mercury process within the biology of the host. Indeed this species has become flattened and almost two-dimensional in its thinness compared to other more helical spirochetes (see next section). The theme within the energy of movement of the spirochetes is communication and transmission of impulses from the higher spiritual realms to the lower material and metabolic realm. The outer flexible bacterial sheath is porous to the influx of these higher energies, whereas the more rigid internal wall holds the geometrical and denser mineralised structure of the material realm (Fig. 12-2). Between the two walls lie the endoflagella that must rotate so as to synchronise and harmonise the signals flowing between the two realms. When this process is disordered then can manifest a syphilitic state of disease, leading to the typical tissue destruction.

Morphology of Treponema pallidum

The Treponema are anaerobic (can survive without oxygen) spirochetes that always require a host animal within which to survive. The best known, Treponema pallidum, differs in appearance from the other spirochetes in having a flat waveform rather than the more usual three-dimensional helical shape. It is a long and yet extremely thin cell, with dimensions of 0.2 by 0.75 micromillimetres diameter and up to 250 micromillimetres in length. It has 6 to 18 spirals and between 2 and 40 endoflagella. Its ends are tapered. Electron microscopy reveals the central axial bundle of the protoplasmic cylinder surrounded by the spiral flagella and the outer sheath membrane.

HOMOEOPATHY OF THE SOLAR SYSTEM: MERCURY

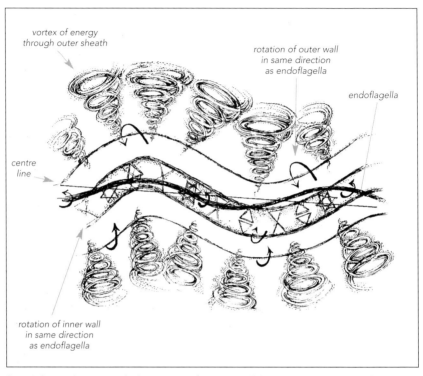

[Fig. 12.2] *Spiritual energies involved in movement of Treponema pallidum at the two walls and endoflagella. There are multi-dimensional and crystalline properties to the energetic radiations from the outer wall.*

It is important to realise that this is not a bacterium that resides in external nature, but is effectively representing a human trait or miasm. It is the microscopic appearance of a distorted energy within the human soul and body. Indeed there are other species of the genus Treponema that are common commensal organisms within the human mouth (at the narrow spaces between the gums and teeth and between the teeth) and perform valuable functions in oral hygiene. These include Treponema denticola, Treponema macrodentium and Treponema oralis. Their functions include the fermentation of amino acids during the oral digestion of protein.

When comparing the shape of the spirochete, specifically Treponema pallidum, there is remarkable similarity with the spiralling serpents around the caduceus of Mercury (see p.83), except that one of the serpents is missing. In effect, syphilis is a one sided distortion of Mercury and the mercurial process. The double helix spiral of two serpents represents the duality of the material realm becoming integrated into unity. It is also the picture of the double helix spirals of two strands of DNA forming a chromosome in the human cell nucleus (Fig. 12-3). One spiral instead of two indicates the one-sided movement of information between the spiritual and material realms; i.e. there is not the integrity between the two planes. Indeed the syphilitic miasm is characterised by one-sided deformity of appearance and behaviour. Thus the face may even appear asymmetrical, and extremes of behaviour can occur, such as mania or depression.

Note there is a close correlation between the symbol of the 'I Ching' (or Chinese Book of Wisdom) with the double helix of chromosomal DNA (or the modern book of life). The ancient Chinese did not use microscopes to probe into the mysteries of life, but could use psychic vision in order to read the etheric realm of formative energy underlying physical events. They drew hexagrams (compositions of six lines) to portray the sixty-four primordial states of energy that they had identified. This is exactly the same as the sixty-four possible sequences of triplet DNA codes (series of three DNA molecules out of a possible four DNA molecule types) that can exist. The ancient Chinese had in fact read the genetic code in its true state as energy, light, colour and sound tones. The 'I Ching' is the same as the human genome; both record the same storage of information within the human gene pool of collective consciousness.

The single coiled serpent is revealed in the staff of Asclepius (the god of healing), which represents the healing journey the soul must undergo to return to the divine mercurial state of communication with the spiritual realm. With this transition the staff develops a double spiral where before there was one. Later, on the soul's journey, a triple phase spiralling energy develops which reflects the forces of trinity within the pranic tube of the initiate. Thus the threefold nature of God

HOMOEOPATHY OF THE SOLAR SYSTEM: MERCURY

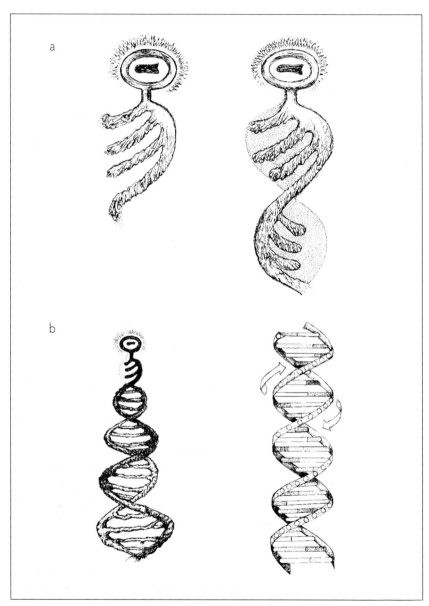

[Fig. 12.3] Symbol for the 'I Ching' compared with chromosomal double stranded DNA: (a) the I Ching symbol appears like the germ of spirit without a physical body; (b) two-stranded DNA arranged as a spiralling ladder with eight cross-links within each 360° spiral. The 'I Ching' symbol neatly fits into the DNA spiral with its four branches.

as Father-Will, Mother-Love and Christ-Wisdom/Child can manifest within the being of the incarnated soul. This is represented in the caduceus by the central rod around which the two serpents are coiled.

The tapered ends of the Treponema pallidum bacterium reveal another block, which the state of syphilis portrays. In the sacred geometry of the double helix or two intertwined spirals, there is no actual end to the spiral. It is a journey into infinity from either end of the structure, representing the infinity of the spiritual and material realms within any potential experience. The spiritual path requires the disciple to leap into the unknown at many points of their journey, when the soul faces the void or the absolute nature of God. It can be terrifying to move past one's comfort zone, but it must be done to clear patterns of dependency in the soul and anchor true co-creativity and the God-spark within. When the ends of the bacterium are tapered it indicates the reticence of the syphilitic state to step beyond this comfort zone of inner experiences. The soul is stagnating within its limited experiences.

An interesting similarity is shown by the telomeres of the chromosomes within the human cell nuclei. The chromosomes are considered to be two-stranded DNA molecules – although they have a twelve stranded DNA nature at subtle spiritual levels. It is beyond the scope of this book to explain this fully, apart from giving a basic overview. The ends of chromosomes are called telomeres and are rather like lace-seals protecting the ends of shoelaces from becoming frayed. Analogously the telomeres protect the ends of the chromosomes from losing vital genetic information every time they replicate with each cell division. It has been found that ageing and cellular death is associated with decay of the telomeres of the chromosomes, whereas immortal cancerous cells have long-lasting telomeres. If the spiritual disciple learns to extend the subtle energy held within each chromosome beyond the confines of the telomeres then in effect the chromosomes no longer stay within a limited pool of information. They can instead act as antennae for channelling from the infinite source of information provided within the cosmic and spiritual realm. The syphilitic bacteria held within the human miasmatic pool then change their ends from tapered to an open-ended array of spirals. They are then able to receive information from the infinite cosmos and shift the human soul from a closed system of energy to one that is open-ended and aligned to its vast and infinitely capable spirit.

That Treponema pallidum is an obligate parasite confirms it is really part of the human psyche and energy field, rather than an external independent entity. Obligate parasite means that it cannot survive alone outside of the human organism. Indeed it is difficult to cultivate it in even in animal tissue. Apart from humans, it can infect apes, rabbits and hamsters in a similar pattern. It rapidly dies if removed from the host body.

Pathogenesis and immunity of syphilis
The initial infection is characterised by an invasion into the body manifesting as an ulcer or sore. There is a local immune and blood vessel response to this invasion, called the primary stage of syphilis. In a later secondary phase, there is a delayed immune response with antibodies produced against the bacteria. One-third of initial patients go onto a tertiary stage when grossly destructive changes occur in various body parts, and it is medically assumed that the antibody immune response is now unable to contain further multiplication and spread of the bacteria.

As in most other chronic infections there are two arms of 'defence' by the immune system: the cellular response and the humoral (antibody) response. The cellular response is the direct attack by lymphocytes, macrophages and other types of white cells to engulf or destroy the bacteria. This can become a delayed response whereby the cells actually start to become hypersensitive despite few bacteria being present, leading to local tissue destruction by local inflammation. The humoral response is the production of several types of antibody with various degrees of specificity towards the bacteria, and thus with varied success at attaching themselves to the bacteria. By doing do the antibodies may be able to de-activate the bacteria, destroy them or at least mark them for the white cells to engulf.

Medical science generally considers the role of the immune system to defend the human organism against invasion and consumption by external pathogenic agents (such as viruses, bacteria, fungi and parasites). The immune system is able to recognise which cells and particles within the body belong to self and which do not. However this is based on a belief system that external microbes are the cause of infections per se. The terrain theory has been suppressed by medical science, but understands rifts in the underlying immune integrity of the body to be the cause of infection. The microbe is instead seen as a normal commensal or inhabitant of the human organism that mutates in the face of the distorted body energy. The microbe is a co-factor in the disease rather than the cause. Thus cure of infection should involve re-integration of the microbe back into a healthy relationship with the human organism. This is a faculty provided by Mercury.

In humanity's ancient past, when souls underwent the fall and separated from the spiritual realm, there arose a stance of duality with the material world. Souls no longer clearly felt their unity with all other life within nature around them. Survival positioning was programmed into the human consciousness, enabling the incarnated beings to feel the illusion of adversity, a harsh environment and the frequent risk of death. If human souls were to incarnate with full mastery and cognisance of their spiritual powers, there would be no sense of the need to evolve or take up challenges in the material realm. These survival programs are particularly evident in the base chakra (the energy centre for grounding and related to adrenal gland function) and the immune system. In Chinese medicine, it is well recognised that wei-chi is a layer of protective energy around the external layers of the body providing a defence against the invasion of external pathogenic factors (including microbes and environmental hazards). The wei-chi is governed by a combination of lung and kidney-adrenal chi. This defence programming within the immune system is now obsolete, for the spiritual journey invokes trust and openness to all other nature kingdoms in the position of unity rather than duality.

When the duality program is released, it enables the true role of the immune system to come forth – which is the ability to communicate with All That Is in an attitude of learning. The immune system then activates certain latent crystalline properties and can communicate with other consciousness beings at other space-time co-ordinates. In effect it becomes a portal for information to flow into and out of the human organism. The absence of a retaliatory reaction to any external information ensures no physical tissue is destroyed in this process of communication. The white cells become memory cells for retaining information and must also be able to release such information in a free flow, so as not to retain obsolete 'immune memory' of past disagreeable experiences. Such experiences would otherwise cause various diseases such as allergies where the body reacts to a memory of the past experience triggered by a similar current experience. Through the influence of Mercury, the past immune memory can be erased (or forgotten) from the white cells, and new information can be gracefully guided into the system.

That past memory of disagreeable experiences can be stored in the old-style immune system is evident also in the mechanism of latency of infection by syphilis. Even though the Treponema pallidum bacteria may exist in very low concentrations, an infected person can re-activate disease many years after the initial infection. It is thought this is due to the bacteria being resident in body sites far removed and therefore protected from the immune system. The bacteria may also have taken up intracellular sites (inside the cells). Tertiary syphilis develops when the bacteria eventually multiply in large numbers again. This process is a sign of retention of the ancient memory of the fall from the spiritual realm with consequent distortion of channelled information. The immune system and body cannot release this disagreeable experience, which is stored as the syphilitic organism itself. Therefore clearing of the syphilitic miasm and syphilitic organism required a release of the memory of the fall within the soul, effectively leading to a re-alignment with the spiritual realm.

This memory *cannot* be cleared by antibiotic treatment, often prescribed in the form of penicillin. It is well known that there is persistence of the bacteria even after high doses of the antibiotic. They especially remain in the cerebrospinal fluid, fluid within the eye (aqueous humour) lymph nodes and nervous system. Notably these are all sites of high ego activity, where the individuality of the human soul must more completely assert itself against foreign invasion.

The syphilitic miasm and bacteria relapses within the general pool of infectious disease in humanity whenever this lesson of separation and distortion from the spiritual realm must be challenged again. It arises whenever significant karmic patterns within human history must be released from collective consciousness. Thus a dramatic pandemic of syphilis occurred at the end of the fifteenth century which decimated many in Europe and Asia. No satisfactory explanation has been made by medical science for the cause of this. However events in the material realm are dependent on causes and intentions from the spiritual realm. At any moment in history there arises the possibility of any new event triggered from the spiritual realm without any relationship with other events in the material realm, even those historically preceding that moment. Thus the reason for the pandemic was the surfacing of ancient Lemurian karma.

Lemuria is the supercontinent preceding Atlantis, and it resonates geographically with the zone of the Pacific Ocean. During Lemuria humanity were still in androgynous (neither male nor female) and displayed fish-like forms. This stage is recapitulated by the first few weeks of the human embryo, when it appears fish-like and the reproductive tissues have not yet differentiated into male or female external genitalia. During mid-Lemuria the human race differentiated into male and female forms, and the blueprints defining masculinity and femininity were relayed from different sectors of the cosmos. This programming of the physical tissues ensured that male and female forms would not be able to 'see' where the other gender had come from. In order words conflict was created between the sexes, providing for an intensification of evolution. If the male and female types within humanity were able to fully understand each other, then no relationship or marital disagreement would be able to occur. This is obviously not the case, and it is probably better for each gender to recognise their incapability to really understand the other half and to come to accept the differences with non-judgement and with grace.

One of the karmic lessons still unresolved from Lemuria is the heightened sexuality that occurred in the human race after the segregation into the two genders. They copulated at an enormous rate, rather like many fish species still do today. However karma was created from the distortion of the proper divine flow of sexual energy, which is actually meant to unite the lower self with the higher self. Sexual energy instead developed cords of sexual dependency, sexual neediness and duality-based relationships between the souls in the promiscuous and unregulated intercourse that occurred. This is the karmic cause of syphilis and the disease became suppressed in Atlantis (for they were unable to heal it).

However it needs to be cleared from the human collective consciousness and with it the syphilitic miasm eventually requires clearing from the human gene pool. This means a re-surfacing of Lemurian consciousness within present humanity, which started actively from the fifteenth century. Thus humanity experienced a worldwide epidemic of the syphilitic disease and over the following centuries fostered a liberation of sacral chakra based sexual energies formerly locked into the Lemurian past. This is flowering now as a heightened sexual awareness between human souls and some of the old Lemurian (and Atlantean karma) is currently being replayed through the promiscuous and distorted sexual behaviour within human society.

Epidemiology of syphilis
By far and away the most usual route for transmitting the bacteria is sexual contact, through body fluids or contact with infected sores on the genitalia. It is uncommon for it to transmit through asexual contact, even when kissing a person with open sores in their mouth. Contaminated blood transfusions can sometimes transmit the bacteria, but after about four days the bacteria is deactivated in stored pooled human blood.

Although the incidence of syphilis as an infection has fallen since the nineteenth century (except for sporadic episodes of increase during war, revolution and large movements of populations geographically) this is merely a suppression of the overtly infectious features of the disease. Instead the late tertiary stages of syphilis have come to the fore as today's common degenerative diseases within the nervous, cardiovascular and skeletal systems.

The modern manifestations of the syphilitic miasm, as suppressed syphilis, are displayed through the following diseases:

- Nervous system – virtually any disease can become expressed, particularly multiple sclerosis, dementia, spinal or cerebellar degeneration and Parkinson's disease.

- Cardiovascular system – again most diseases are syphilitic, especially aortic aneurysm (dilatation of the aorta in thoracic or abdominal regions), aortic dissection (a tear within the aorta wall with blood tracking into the wall), heart valve disorders of all types (e.g. aortic valve stenosis and narrowing) and coronary artery disease.

- Skeletal system – most deforming degenerative disorders here are syphilitic, often with sycotic miasmatic features (the miasm of suppressed gonorrhoea). Those particularly syphilitic are osteoporosis, Pagets disease (an overgrowth of the bone), psoriatic deforming arthritis, rheumatoid arthritis and rickets.

This suppression of syphilis would require appropriate remedies to bring the miasm up the surface and thereafter be cleared. Homoeopathic Mercury is a key remedy in this regard, bearing in mind until only recently the excessive use of material and toxic doses of metallic Mercury to treat (but consequently suppress) syphilis.

There has been a recent increase in syphilis (especially neuro-syphilis) in the Western world due largely to an increased rate of infection by the HIV virus in homosexual men, intravenous drug users and their sexual partners with co-incidental infection with syphilis. In the AIDs (acquired immuno-deficiency syndrome) stage of HIV infection the past syphilitic infection also re-activates with disastrous consequences. In the third world, notably in Asia and Africa, there is also an increase of syphilis in heterosexual groups with HIV infection, especially spread through prostitution. Again much of this is the surfacing of old Lemurian karma between human souls, distorting their sacral and sexual centres with disease.

The features of late stage or tertiary syphilis have become less clear cut and more difficult to diagnose on clinical grounds. This is partly due to the suppression by drugs in the high-risk groups, especially antibiotics, which distort the immune response, and also by vaccinations.

Chapter 13

Mercury in breathing and circulation

The formation of the lungs involves the energy of Mercury. Mercury as messenger of the gods mediates between heaven and Earth. The metal Mercury mediates the cosmic realm with the mineral kingdom. Similarly in the lungs, the soul-spiritual being of the human mediates with its Earth being.

Inspiration/inhalation

Breathing acts as a powerful multidimensional arena for the flow of consciousness, especially in the astral body. There is an awareness of subtle energy and light within pathways for the flow of consciousness, with each inbreath being a representation of the creative breath of the Source in manifesting All That Is. With each inspiration comes an increase of consciousness, which allows many other beings across time and space to be made available to the self. Oxygen allows an infusion of spirit and will-oriented energy to vitalise the creation of substance, be it another being, planet or star system. Each inspiration provides prana to create something. Oxygen as such is not a gas devoid of any upper dimensional awareness; indeed every individual will oxygenate their system in unique ways, depending on how plastic and flexible the lungs are in co-ordinating the transmissions of oxygen to the rest of one's beingness.

Exhalation

By exhaling carbon dioxide (CO_2) the self is reaffirming and constantly creating a base on the planet. Carbon dioxide is a product of a grounded perspective on Earth, and is a substance made from Earth material, to be released into the air element. This carbon dioxide

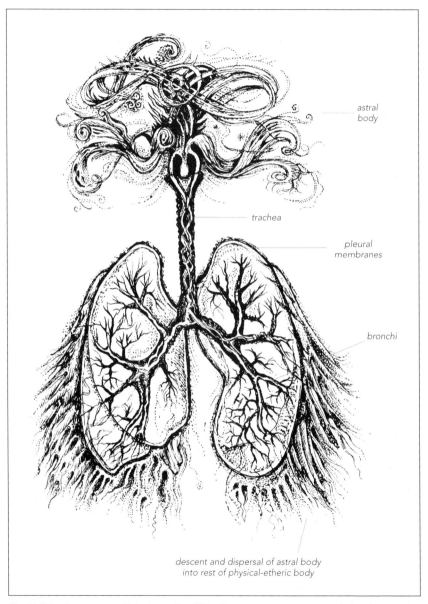

[Fig. 13.1] *Respiratory system with depiction of astral flow. The upper respiratory airways as pharynx, larynx, trachea and two main bronchi. The lungs further divide into smaller bronchi until terminal bronchioles end with alveoli. The movement of the astral body is shown, as a rhythmic partial entry into and out of the lungs.*

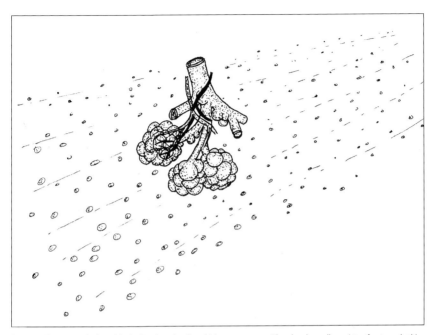

[Fig. 13.2] *Portion of a lung lobule showing alveoli and Mercury process. The alveolar wall consists of extremely thin epithelial cells, providing a thin barrier to gas exchange.*

originated as material carbohydrate and carbon-based substance within the planet. Exhalation and the metabolic reactions preceding the formation of carbon dioxide represent the conversion of something ponderable and material in Earth (earthly carbon) into something imponderable and immaterial (carbon dioxide gas into the atmosphere). Each expiration allows oneself to stabilise, change or shape the plant and etheric realms on the planet across time and space, providing a fluid basis from which conscious evolution can proceed. The self can alter all the beings that have existed on the planet simply by altering the way the carbon dioxide formed in the body is released.

Astral body incarnation and the state of soul

The lungs provide for the entry of the air organism and through this process the human is intensely and more consciously connected with the environment. Part of the air of the environment becomes the inner world for a moment and inside the physical body. This contact with the environment is more intensive, although more subtle, than the interaction through the gastrointestinal tract of food from the environment. The lungs provide a surface exquisitely open to the environment (Fig. 13-1). Also the formation of hollow spaces or invagination of tissue (which occurs in lung formation to form tubular alveoli) is an astral process (Fig. 13-2). It is the astral body that, by moving into the physical-etheric tissues of the embryo, provides the driving force for the formation of hollowed tubes making up the lungs. Through the lungs, the astral body incarnates.

The lungs are not merely supplying the body with oxygen and expelling carbon dioxide. If this were their only purpose then they would be actually very inefficient at it. For example, the gaseous exchange in the gills of fish is much more effective than that in humans. Over and above a physiological process there is a higher function involved in the lungs. Human and animal respiration is the reverse of plant respiration; it is an oxidation process rather than a reduction. Humans forms air (carbon dioxide) from the substance of their body, i.e. from the earthly nature of the body. Thus solid substance is freed and life force is transformed through breathing – into metabolic light and warmth. Through breathing there is a brief stoppage in the stream of breath, between out- and in- breathing.

In terms of anthroposophical-oriented medicine the rhythmic system (heart and lungs) provides the basis for the feeling life. Conversely the nervous and sensory system is the basis for the thinking life and the metabolic system the basis for the life of will. Soul perceptions can be brought about by a damming up process within the physical body, such as damming up the blood by stopping its stream, or damming up the breath by the pause between in and out breaths. Indeed many yogic techniques involve breath-holding techniques. There is an interaction between feeling and the rhythm of breathing, such as the change in breathing rate when excited or fearful, or deep breathing during the release of tension or depression. The breathing rate gives an indication of the person's state of soul. By transiently stopping the breath the soul has the opportunity to provide the force for feeling.

The lungs therefore rule the dissolving and densification of substance by the soul-spiritual being anchoring to its earthly body. Thus it is the first breath and not the actual exit of the baby's physical body from the maternal vagina at birth that is the beginning of the present incarnation on Earth. This beginning is not the same as the vegetative life that starts in the etheric body of the embryo within the womb, before birth. It is only actual breathing by the newborn baby that makes possible the higher impulses of the soul-spirit and the astral body to come into activity within the physical body. Thus the lungs by their structure enable the incarnation process of the soul and astral body. The lungs regulate the relationship of the soul to the physical body.

The lungs are specially related to the heart and the kidneys. Through the lungs the astral body and the dynamics of the nervous system are intense. Through the heart there is more a relationship to the blood system orientated towards the metabolic system. Between the heart and lungs there is the dynamic relationship with a ratio of respiration to the pulse of 4:1, and both form the rhythmic system as the structural basis of the feeling life. The kidneys are the organs that regulate the breathing through of the organism. Lungs and kidneys are both astral organs where lungs are the performing and kidneys are the ruling organs of breathing.

The lungs take in prana as well as oxygen. Indeed the intake and flow of prana is the primary function in a spiritual context. Prana enters directly into the etheric body with each breath and distributes to the various centres of the body. Any misuse of energy will tend to pre-dispose the lungs to illness. Karmic consequences of past life actions with a misuse of energy can lead to defects of lungs in this incarnation either from birth or a pre-disposition to disease during life with illnesses such as tuberculosis, bronchitis, pneumonia or asthma. By experiencing shortness of breath the individual will remember at a subconscious level that they once misused energy and will resolve never to do so again. Allergies within the lungs also often relate to the misuse of energy. In some cases the energy can arise from a traumatic experience from present or past lives: thus most cat allergies are due to the sufferer having once been killed or mauled by some member of the cat family. This memory within the astral body, even though stemming from a past life, is working into the lungs of the present life. Thus a panic attack of the soul and astral body occurs when it meets a member of the cat family again, in case the former negative experience is repeated. This panic attack is experienced physically as an asthmatic attack, rather than mentally as a panic attack, due to the veil of consciousness clouding the source of the problem from the conscious mind.

Mercury helped to program the physical body with this polarity and rhythm of death and life forces. Thus the inspiration of the astral body through inhalation of air required the vibration of Mercury within the lungs to receive this wakefulness or consciousness of the material world, and thus the sensation of being alive. The exhalation of stale air as waste products of cellular respiration is actually a flowing out of the astral body from the physical, and with it a movement of this subtle body back towards the spiritual realm whence it came. This came to represent the process of death, i.e. when death occurs the soul completely leaves the physical body and fully breaks the link between this and the astral and higher subtle bodies. For many souls their astral body still retains a memory of the death process at the end of their past lives, but they often react with fear and panic if such a déjà vu re-experience occurs during this lifetime.

Thus Mercury can balance the death and life forces within the human physiology again. It enables incorporation of the proper blueprints into the physical-etheric tissues by channelling these appropriately from the higher subtle bodies of astral, mental and spiritual bodies and under the guidance of spirit or the higher self. A sense of self or I-ness can thus incorporate right into the physical cells. Homoeopathic Mercury, being its material counterpart, is excellent for restructuring tissues stuck in chronic or recurrent infection and inflammation. It guides the incorporation of new and healthy blueprints that should be in that region of tissue and thus assist healthy regeneration of the area.

Mercury and iron forces

Iron (and its related Mars forces) facilitates the action of Mercury within the human physiology. The whole act of breathing is deeply connected to iron. Oxygen intake and exchange requires red blood cell haemoglobin in which iron is active. The process of incarnation also requires iron. Inhalation and exhalation mirrors the whole process of breakdown or oxidation and excretion on the one side and build-up of body substance and growth on the other side. Through breathing the ego (sense of self) of the human enters a connection with the physical world and at the same time has an experience of the spiritual world. In and out breathing allows wakefulness in the physical world and also awakening in the spirit. Connecting with the Earth requires the individual coming into the Earth and grasping corporeality. This also involves taking hold of oneself through the limbs and the development of the limbs is connected with the development of the lungs and the breathing process.

The first breath of the newborn baby is an act of breakdown, a catabolic process with oxidation. There is indeed temporarily a decrease of the body weight after birth and this is the breakdown of the old motherly-derived body substance, which is breathed out and excreted (partly as carbon dioxide) to allow space for the building up of new individual body substance. The burning up of brown fat stores in the newborn activates the warmth process and thus the ego incarnates more strongly. Many babies are, however, being forcefully incarnated through infertility treatments to aid conception (such as in vitro fertilisation), as well as through excessive use of iron supplements during pregnancy.

The spiritual significance of human blood

An understanding of the spiritual significance of breathing also requires an understanding of the role played by the heart and blood circulation. The blood, as for all other human organs and tissues, has undergone huge transformations during the evolution of humanity – and more changes are to come. In the ancient past, when humans lived within an etheric material realm, the world was not as hard, dense and mineralised. Their blood was not red, as it is now, but a white ethereal fluid similar to milky-white plant juice. The body of the human was attached to the etheric body of the Earth rather like an unborn baby to the placenta by an umbilical cord. The milky energy was fed to humans through etheric umbilical cords from the Earth.

However, when humans densified further into harder physical bodies, the blood changed colour to red. The Lords of Form under the constellation of Scorpio had fashioned the physical body into the present form, and the fiery Angels of Mars then used the iron on Earth to incorporate the fire and iron forces into the blood. This was done to enable human egos (through the element of warmth) to become incorporated into the blood, and thereby anchor into the body the capacity for reincarnation and personal freedom. Thus the human became dimly aware of its 'I' nature.

In the past human sacrifices and the spilling of blood was an important part of religious culture and most victims volunteered willingly. Examples can be seen in various Pacific Sea island races (such as Bali), the South American Mayans, Aztecs and Incas. These civilisations knew of the afterlife and death was not looked upon as the end. Individual spiritual progress was much accelerated by the spilt blood flowing back into the electromagnetic fields of Earth. The blood would flow through the soul's influence to all people and situations that were connected with it, especially to those the body had been sacrificed. The sacrificed could sense angelic beings ready to escort their passage into the spiritual realm, and so were not afraid. Similarly humanity has chosen to spill and flow blood at a mass level during war and battle, in an attempt to dissolve cultural and racial prejudices and boundaries. By spilling blood on foreign soil the soldier would ethereally create a relationship with that land, overcoming any former alienation from it.

The arterial blood carries fresh forces of prana and vitality to the tissues, and the venous blood carries the obsolete and past-oriented information from the body to be released into the lungs. Blood is a medium for the ego to exert itself in the physical body. That mature red blood cells do not contain nuclei whilst in circulation allows freedom for the ego, for the red blood cells are then not susceptible to influence or regulation by outside forces. They can also reflect the path of the soul through its many incarnations, each phase having a veil of ignorance and unconsciousness between them, which allows a truer concept of freedom through uncertainty. A hypnotist is actually pushing out the ego consciousness of the individual in order to influence the lesser mind and desire/emotional mind of the person with the hypnotist's agenda. This makes the blood and lower personality less under the control of one's own ego. The red blood cells in this situation then become nucleated, since nuclei allow outside forces to influence the cells. The blood also becomes denser and prevents the person's own ego from penetrating it, thus allowing the outside ego forces to take over.

Part of any spiritual development is the transformation of the Saturn-ruled skeleton with a Jupiter influence and involves the activation of the bone marrow to spiritualise the blood even more. The blood assists in the alchemical process of spiritualising the skeleton, as it is actually a very refined light-filled essence. The more spiritualised a person becomes, the more the blood becomes rarefied and less heavy. Saints have been known to have white blood and a buoyant radiant body.

Purification of the blood includes dietary practices to avoid thickening the blood with excess or impure foods (especially prohibiting consumption of meat containing the suffering of animals). The misuse of the creative forces within the body, the use of tamasic or impure foods, lowly thought and speech all tend to thicken the blood. The future race of humanity will not however inhabit as dense a physical body.

The red blood also has a special relationship to the astral body whose evolution began in the third creative day (Moon period) of the present Earth chain (see p.36). Circulation appeared at that time (i.e. start of fluid forces); initially the blood was white and influenced by desire forms. The luciferic beings then concentrated the red ray into the blood to further stimulate the passions and desire forces. Red blood allows for animalistic emotions and the human ego must learn to take hold of these red blood cells as part of its control over the lower desire nature. In this way the red cells attract more fire forces of the Earth and Sun as part of the oxygenation process. White blood cells are germ centres and are linked to negative and destructive thought processes, which must be transformed to overcome the negative forces of vulnerability, hostility to the outside world and survival programming.

The red blood cells of animals contain a nucleus, which is not found within human red cells. This is the centre through which the group animal spirit controls the species. During human embryonic life, the foetal red cells also contain nuclei to allow the mother to exert influence over its growth, and these disappear after birth to allow the child's own ego to take over. When there is control of the person by another ego, as in uncontrolled mediumship, overpowering control or in obsession, the red cells become nucleated again.

Today the marriage between people of different races and cultures allows the ego forces to mix into unity. However in the past the strict customs of marrying only within the family, such as between cousins or within the tribe or culture, strengthened the ties between the egos of the families. This made it easier to impress upon the subconscious minds of family members their ancestral traditions with least distortion. In this way family and tribal instincts were developed and preserved through the generations, which would later allow the egos' to take up the race characteristics at a spirit level.

International and cross-cultural marriage allows the breaking of racial egotism – breaking down stuck perspectives and having a crystallising effect on the blood. At present the blood of an individual contains pictures of their own personal experiences which are accessed through the subconscious mind. Humans typically govern their lives in accordance to the pictures stored within the blood. Familiarity with certain behaviours can make a person tolerant to them, as in violence or vice. During the time of marriage within the family, individuals were ruled by a family spirit or angel, which entered the body through inhaled air and helped the person's ego control its vehicle. When cross cultural and marriage outside the family started, the egos had reached the level of evolution when they no longer depended on these outside forces and could start guiding from within as co-creators. The more the blood is mixed with ego forces of others the less influenced is the person's own ego by the family spirit/angel. Thus human blood became more and more mixed.

Unmixed blood allowed the ancestral forces to govern the individual, but would now give a negative clairvoyance of the latent pictures within the blood. Mixed blood allowed the power of personal experience and positive clairvoyance with freedom from ancestral ties.

If the soul is forcefully wrenched out of the physical body (as in violent death), the impure vibrations in the lower nature that are stored in the venous blood cling to the departing ego. If the blood is allowed to flow these are cleansed out of the system and the ego feels a proper liberation from the physical body.

Heart and lung circulation

From the heart, blood is sent to be of use to all parts of the body, carrying nutritive energy and fresh information from the spiritual realm. Each stream of venous blood returning from the periphery toward the heart carries its own unique experience. From the liver comes a stream of purified blood laden with carbohydrate sugars and nutritive substance gathered from the digestive tract via the portal vein. The finest venous blood comes from the head centres with its spiritual infusion of thought-forms into the blood. Energetically more exhausted venous blood returns from the limbs and muscles of the whole body with the experience of labour and exertion. The various venous channels thus bring different mixtures of vibrations and materials, each with their particular cleansing role, to the heart.

The heart must prepare and eject vitalised arterial blood that is able to disseminate energy into all regions of the body. The heart requires the lungs to purify the venous blood of those toxins and experiences that are obsolete within the bloodstream. The lungs therefore act to discern every particle of blood that they receive. The pulmonary arteries divide into capillaries that supply the walls of the air chambers (alveoli) within the lungs. Using the spiritual faculties of wisdom and discernment the pulmonary membranes attune to the qualities of the blood. These membranes guide the venous blood in releasing those foul and materially gross gases and vapours that need expelling, passing these out into the general atmosphere. Oxygen and other vapours are absorbed to enrich the blood. The blood returns from the lungs through the pulmonary veins to the left side the heart, brighter in colour, livelier in motion and less gross.

It is then projected to the body, not as an unwilling sluggish stream, but with an elastic and enthusiastic bound into every gland, cell and muscle fibre in the body. Every part of the body in various ways indicates its requirements to the arterial bloodstream. The heart imbues the arterial stream with many new spiritual vibrations eager for expression in the physical body. The blood has a consciousness that draws the necessary elements towards the organ that needs it most. Thus the finest most purified blood ascends to the head; the streams rich in astral power flow to the muscles of the body and limbs; the more sluggish earthly blood descends to the spleen; and poor quality blood to the kidneys for removal of chemical toxic waste.

The rhythmic breathing of the lungs moves the ribs and diaphragm and through these the whole viscera, muscles and every cell of the body has motion dependent on the lungs. Similarly the motion of the heart connects to all the cells of the body. Angels are in constant attendance within the human energy field, anchoring divine sacred geometries into the expression of the physical body. The spiritual heart continually inspires unconditional love, and the breathing action of the spiritual lungs constantly interprets this love, enabling the dispersion and radiance of this love. The heart supplies blood at the pressure through which every body part can be filled and the lungs provide the sheathing of this blood with pranic energy. There is an internal respiratory rhythm within the spiritual realm, which cannot be perceived normally, flowing into the human external respiration.

Without this subtle rhythmic pulse a human would instantly die and the same applies to a spiritual beating of the heart.

In the spiritual world, a soul's faith is known by its breathing cycle and a soul's compassionate love by the beating of its heart. Although a human is capable of a selfish and materialistic life, inner development improves truthfulness of the thinking and opens the heart to greater love. Wisdom cleanses this love from its lower gross nature and introduces it to spiritual expression. This is similar to the purification of the coarse deoxygenated blood by the lungs. Blood flows from the heart into the lungs in greater abundance than it flows back from the lungs into the heart. It enters the lungs undigested and impure, but returns refined and pure. Within the lungs the blood is purified and its useless particles released as vapour for exhalation. The heart anchors love and will and the lungs provide perception of thought and understanding, by which purification can occur.

Through the lungs, a worldly human can become spiritual and celestial by nourishing the soul. The atmosphere is full of volatile elements and odours as well as numerous frequencies of spirit. There are some airy elements that are injurious to the soul and some that nurture it. By closing to wisdom and preferring gross thoughts, the lungs inhale those dense odours corresponding to such thoughts. This fouls the blood. The angels take delight in channelling those elements corresponding to love and wisdom, whereas demons in hell take delight only in the elements that correspond with lust and stupidity. Humans impregnate their blood with such things according to how their love and discernment flow. It is the role of Mercury to assist the whole process of detoxification within the lungs, and to guide new spiritual currents into the blood.

Chapter 14

Occult anatomy and the hermaphrodite nature

The Mercury process is important for proper nerve cell function. It influences the movement of thoughts within the central nervous system, with widespread effects on personality development and memory. It is also important for gender differentiation of the brain tissues.

The meninges (surface sheaths) of the brain are important for electrical balance in the underlying nerve tissue. The pia mater represents the delicate innermost lining of the meninges around the brain and spinal cord. Pia is the feminine of 'pious', meaning 'godly' or being devoted to deity, while mater means 'mother'. Thus pia mater is the Holy Mother, containing within herself the foetus of the heavenly human. Mater is a word used in connection to the origin or source of the gods.

The heavenly human is androgynous, the foetus within the Divine Mother that is hermaphrodite, having both male and female parts. This dual nature can be seen within the brain. For example a structure called the corpora quadrigemina with four rounded tissues lies immediately behind the third ventricle. It is esoterically under the control of Saturn. Of the four masses the anterior pair is called the nates or buttocks and the posterior pair called the testes. Near the corpora quadrigemina are two further rounded lumps called the mammillary bodies, so called because they look like two small breasts. The names for these structures reflect their similar appearance to reproductive parts, with the existence of parts derived from both male and female systems found next to each other in this region of the brain.

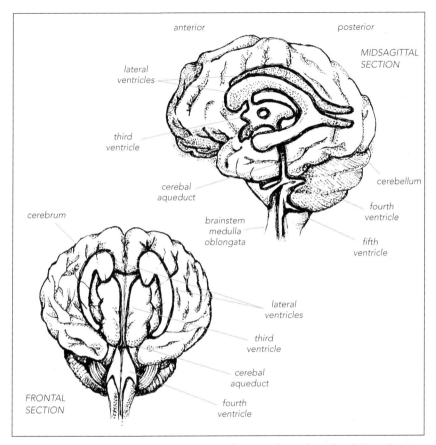

[Fig. 14.1] *Cerebrum and brainstem. The cerebrum consists of two cerebral hemispheres. Convulations and grooves make up the surface appearance. Within the brain lies a complex system of cavities containing cerebrospinal fluid, the ventricular system. The brainstem is the portion connecting the cerebral hemispheres to the spinal cord.*

Thus the brain reflects the androgynous nature of the being. Also, the pineal and pituitary glands are the generative organs of this celestial hermaphrodite. The pineal gland corresponds to the uterus in the female and the penis in the male. The pituitary gland corresponds to the breasts in the female. The hermaphrodite being is capable of being male and female, of being its own mother and father. The brain is thus two beings, locked within an embrace like twins within the womb. This further reveals the influence of Gemini, the twins, symbolising Adam and Eve before the separation. The brain is also similar in appearance to the spermatozoon, or sperm cell. The coiled-up head within the sperm is reflective of the future brain the embryo will have.

The brain and reproductive organs

There is a close connection between the brain and the reproductive organs. The brain (Fig. 14-1) and larynx were built out of conserved creative sexual force, for sexual energy is creative no matter where it is used. By conserving and transmuting sexual energy, the human can create beautiful forms. The sacred fire when lifted into the brain is not passion but light and heralds the new race of humanity. The organs of physical procreation will then atrophy and their function taken over by the larynx, heart and brain, so creation will be through verbal and thinking activity, by projection and materialisation of images. Great spiritual adepts can create physical bodies for themselves out of cosmic substance through their own will and imagination, thus having mastery over life and death. The intimate link between the brain and creative organs is shown in that excessive abuse of the sex drive will weaken the nerves and brain, for both draw on the same energy for their functioning.

The fiery kundalini serpent energy lies coiled within the base chakra and has a link to the cerebrum. During the early development of the human being, fire forces descended from the brain centres in order to create the kundalini in the base. The spiritual initiate awakens this force to lead it back up to the brain, not simply by physical chastity of sex, but by the chastity of the soul (when human no longer finds pleasure in vice). In fact negative abstinence when the lower lust based sexual nature has not been transformed but instead suppressed can do more harm than good.

The sacrum is triangular in shape and symbolises the sacred altar of the temple, close to the sleeping serpent power. When awakened this power can be sacrificed in order to spiritualise the gross elements so as to lift the fire. Humans normally drag this power downward in opposition to the celestial/divine. Here is the inner reflection of the external world's religious burnt offerings and altars of purification. When this fire reaches the pineal gland then human and spiritual become united. The initiate must then learn to overcome the urges of the lower nature by focusing on creating higher forms of activity (e.g. by higher thoughts, divine images, spiritualised outer activities) in order to channel this fire wisely. Meditation on divine forms will transform the sexual and etheric energies into energy for the heart and brain.

The blending of the two nervous systems will make the human both male and female. The brain contains both male and female parts. The initiate will unite the forces of Hermes and Aphrodites, to become hermaphrodite. This union has a marriage altar in the larynx. The spiritual evolution in Lemuria and Atlantis was along the feminine lines of force; when many of the spiritual leaders incarnated into female bodies. During that time period most humans lived largely through their brainstem, spinal cord and involuntary nervous system. The present human race has to deal with masculine forces and the voluntary nervous system, until there is final blending of the two polarities of gender.

Past occult practices used during Lemuria and Atlantis, including trance mediumship (whereby dreamlike images were brought up from the sympathetic nervous system), are no longer valid. With such techniques, clairvoyant powers develop whereby images of distant events in the material world can be brought up in hypnotic states. This was the way the outer world was contacted in Lemuria, especially under the guidance of luciferic spirits who used women as the subjects. During Atlantis, consciousness was shifted from the inner to the outer planes, to achieve the present objective externalised consciousness. The soul now learns to consciously use the brain centres and remain whole so as to anchor the I Am Presence within.

The human has two bodies, one fashioned from the elements and the other from the stars, and there are two nervous systems at present. These two were made under the supervision of the Lords of Form at the zodiacal hierarchy of Scorpio. Mercury as the hierarchical planetary ruler of Scorpio (see p.74) guides this information into the embryonic tissues of the human nervous system.

The root races and procreation

As within the current fourth chain of Earth's evolution (see p.36) the present population is the fifth root race. The root races can be studied to understand reproductive development on Earth. Before the root races there existed pure spiritual consciousness as projected by the spiritual will and law of the Creator. This is the dawning of the rebirth of a world and is called the seed Manu.

The first root race was the self-born and existed as astral shadows of their progenitors. The body under development had no understanding of mind, intelligence or will. The inner spiritual being, self or monad was unconnected to the body. The link had not yet been made between spirit and matter.

From this first root race emanated the second root race called the sweat born or the bone-less. The theme here was the development of solar energy, light and nourishment and the ability to feed from the substance of the material world. Some of the beings here are called Rakshasas (also termed demons and preservers and who were required to feed on other beings) plus the incarnating gods (Asuras and Kumaras). There was the first primitive and weak spark of intelligence as spirit within matter. One of the early methods of procreation was the evolution of one's image through drops of sweat, which would be seen as magic now. But these early second root race beings were able to ooze another being out of their own bodies. This has been seen in mediums who can ooze out of their own body various energies from the spiritual world. This is also an allegory of the genesis of Adam born as an image of clay into which the Lord God breathes the life breath. It does not however provide for the intellect or discrimination that he had to develop subsequent to tasting the fruit of the tree of knowledge.

The third root race was the androgynous beings. The initial sub races were shells and conscious beings later who inhabited their bodies. Initially they were without gender and evolved out of themselves. Later they became oviparous: they secreted emanations from their bodies as spherical nuclei that developed into large soft egg-like vehicles. These eggs gradually hardened and, after a period of gestation, broke to release their young. Thus the early humans laid eggs.

Thus a progressive order of the methods of reproduction can be listed:

- Fission. This is initially the division of a homogeneous speck of the cell such as the amoeba, which divides into two. The nucleus of the cell splits into two similar nuclei which then develop within the same cell wall or break it to become two independent cells. This relates to the first root race.

- Budding. Here a small portion of the original organism swells out of its surface and finally parts company to form a bud, which will eventually grow to the size of the original being. This still occurs in many vegetables. It relates to the reproduction methods of the second root race.

- Spores. Here a single cell is thrown off from the parent organism, which develops into a multi-cellular organism having features similar to the parent. This still occurs in bacteria and mosses.

- Intermediate hermaphrodites. Here male and female organs are in the same individual and this still occurs in most plants, worms and snails. It is related to the second and early third root races.

- True sexual union. This developed in the later third root race. The sons of wisdom (also called the spiritual dhyanis) had become intellectual enough through their contact with matter during previous cycles of incarnation to allow them to become independent self-conscious entities in the material plane. Through their karma and incarnation they acquired enough experience to become ready. They became the sages or arhats.

In this third root race the Lemurian beings included towering giants of great strength and beauty. However they also represented the fallen race that fell to matter. The main gods and heroes of the fourth and fifth root races (Atlantis and the current human race respectively) are based on memories of these beings from the third root race. These beings had a dual nature for they had great virtue and godliness and yet also fell to great sin. This is the race preceding Adam and Eve. They developed the power with which to create duality and male and female forms. This mysterious and divine creative power is latent in the will and energy of every human but only becomes developed by the highest spiritual training, being presently dormant in the vast majority of humans. The third root race created the sons of will and yoga, the spiritual forefathers or ancestors of the subsequent masters and arhats.

In the early third root race the method of procreation changed. The drops of sweat became even greater drops, which expanded into large ovoid bodies or huge eggs. In these the human foetus gestated for several years. The race then developed into the early Lemurian androgynous and hermaphrodite race. The form these Lemurians took was typically rounded, having the back and sides as of a circle and great force and strength. Spiritual hierarchy and the gods divided them into two, i.e. to create the male and female forms over a long period of time. Initially reproduction was by creating buds and polyps. Later eggs were more developed. Note that laws of karma override the tendencies of hereditary.

During the initial separation and development of gender types there were beings created with both male and female forms. Initially one gender would predominate over the other in an individual person, until that person became more fully male or female. The egg cells and the babies were also developed with both male and female forms. There was still mostly a dreamy collective consciousness within the beings. As the beings became unisexual or male and female forms separated, this created tension between the two genders. This conflict has been very important for the further development of the human race. It also created a denser and more grounded reality and allowed the development of the denser more mineralised Earth. Babies were becoming more like modern-day babies and lost the faculty of walking as soon as they were liberated from their shell. Thus by the end of the fifth sub race (of seven) within the Lemurian chain, humanity was under similar reproductive states as they are now.

The Lemurians were horticultural and worked closely with the plant kingdom. Their influence is demonstrated by the majority of plants still having both male and female forms within their flowers, with the ability to self-pollinate a seed for the next generation. Dual sexuality is also displayed in many lower animals. Indeed in the growth of the human embryo, the distinction of gender does not happen until a considerable time has elapsed.

Syphilis and the Lemurian age

The Lemurian age preceding the Atlantean age roughly existed one billion years ago, although linear third-dimensional time is not an accurate measure for the history of the planet. During the early Lemurian segregation into the two genders, Mercury played a part in relaying the required blueprints for male and female body development. These codes came from different parts of the cosmos. This gender development facilitated proper evolution of the human species by providing scope for conflict and evolutionary interplay between the two halves of the human race. Although a particular soul can reincarnate as female in one life, and male in the next, still the fact remains that the female and male divisions cannot fully understand the codes programming the other gender type (since they come from separate and very different parts of the cosmos). This generated feelings such as excitement at discovery of the gifts of the other gender type, as well as the feeling of love and attraction for that which is different and opposite to oneself. In the initial separation however, during early Lemuria, there was not the more conscious emotional awareness of sexuality that we have now.

Just before the gender separation, the beings could best be described as gel and amoeboid like, without secondary sexual characteristics. The division created a fish like body, as yet with very limited distinct features defining the sexes. However sexual behaviour had now begun, as symbolised by the reproductive awareness of Adam and Eve in the garden of Eden. In fact this led to uncontrolled heightened sexuality. Beings copulated with each other without any particular sense of the commitment or morality that we would aspire to now. It would even have appeared to us as the extreme of promiscuity and frenzied coitus, and included beings related to each other. They copulated even whilst giving birth to their children. The more advanced aspired to a committed relationship with each other, but this was a minority. This behaviour was a consequence of the separation from the spiritual realm (the fall) for there was much less ethos encoded naturally into material life.

The karmic consequence of all this sexuality was the disease of syphilis (see p.153). It created the syphilitic miasm within the human gene and consciousness pool. Syphilis represents the auto-destructive processes engendered by a lack of ethos and morality through the separation from the spiritual plane. It will be found that all miasms are in some shape or form a consequence of the separation of the lower self and the human species from the spiritual realm. The miasm of syphilis is however particular to a self-destructive process. Death was also now programmed into humanity, as a tool for returning back to the spiritual realm after a lifetime on Earth. The length of this Lemurian lifetime was extremely long compared to the standard modern human life (although there are many humans on Earth who have lived thousands of years). During Lemuria and until quite recent post-Atlantean times, humanity understood death not to be the complete end of existence. It was perceived to an extent that the human soul lived on. Indeed for early humanity death was welcomed when opportune, for it meant a return to the lap of the gods and a renewal of spiritual forces within the soul matrix.

As shown by the staff of Mercury, the double coiled caduceus (see p.83), a property of Mercury is to heal rifts in the spiralling energy within the spinal cord. The relevance this has for syphilis can now be discussed. Another perspective of syphilis is as a disease of excessive and unregulated sex and breeding between peoples of different races and cultures. This is not, however, a morally derogatory statement. The human soul has experiences within multiple cultures and races over its long biography. A problem can arise however when a person's blood codes cannot mix well with the codes of another person after union of energies through sexual intercourse. This is especially a problem if more spiritually and culturally advanced races interbreed with primitive races, which happened many times over human history. The blood contains unique blueprints to do with the essential ego character of that person.

Syphilis arises when contrasting and foreign bloodstreams mix together. Mixed inappropriately it causes an abnormal spiralling of the electrical, magnetic and gravitational waveforms within the blood and the related nervous energy in the pranic tube of the spinal cord. Holes appear in this pranic tube from the sexual cords linking the person to not only their sexual partner, but also to all this partner's other partners. When the sexual centres are under weak guidance from the head chakras, then cords of etheric and astral substance link all the sexual partners throughout the time-space and incarnation grid that have any common partners amongst them. This creates an enormous orgiastic matrix of sexual energy. It can initially seem exciting for a soul to experience such heightened and multiple sexual incidents and with so many partners at subtle levels of consciousness, but ultimately the immense amount of sexual energy generated becomes stuck in the physical and etheric bodies. The multiple sexual experiences create disease at etheric and lower astral realms, which on the physical plane of reality has become the condition known as syphilis. It is due to the breakdown of the lesser ego or personality as it becomes bombarded and affected by myriad and unhealthy sexual cords. This condition then becomes contagious and passed onto further sexual partners, simply by etherically linking that partner into the matrix of sexual energy just described. Syphilis also requires a breach in the skin for the contagion or bacterium to pass through to the next partner. This reveals another aspect – for it is the weakness of the ego or character forces which enables syphilis to infect the organism. This character weakness causes a rift in the defence layer of etheric energy around the body, for there is a lack of integrity of self versus non-self.

The ancients learnt of medicines empirically through direct observation of nature. They studied more than simply those substances found on Earth, but also the relationships between stellar bodies and disease prevalence. They noticed that certain diseases had a worse prognosis at certain transits of the solar system planets, and that a generally poorer prognosis prevailed when the malefic planet pertaining to that disease was above the Earth horizon. An improved prognosis resulted from descent of that planet below the horizon of Earth. They thus discovered the powerful influence the planet Mercury had on the progression of syphilis in a patient. When Mercury was above the horizon, the prognosis was poor and the patient more likely to die. They then discovered that mineral and organic forms of Mercury could counteract this influence of planetary Mercury. It was as if the patient used the internalised Mercury to strengthen him/herself against the oppression of planetary Mercury. This is remarkably close to the homoeopathic principle of treating like with like. The ancients also knew how to ameliorate the toxic effects of mineral Mercury as a medicament. They found that plants and animal-based medicines rich in Mercury were effective but without the toxicity. Such plants and animals were invariably found in the vicinity of Mercury mines, and were due to the organism absorbing the Mercury substance from the soil and into the tissues. Thus it was plants with strong root systems and animals that live predominantly underground that were most efficacious. Salamanders and toads were amongst the animal remedies, and these are considered to be mercurial animals.

Sexual energy distortions

Sexual energy is a union between various aspects of one's being. This occurs at multiple levels, as follows:

- The union between spirit and matter and is thus the attractive force inviting the lower self within the material realm to connect to the evolutionary energy of return to Spirit. It is the union between life and form.

- It is the urge that draws man to woman for the purpose of procreation of new life forms, to provide the physical bodies for another incarnating soul.

- Sex is an outer manifestation of an inner spiritual reality. This inner reality is that of the relationship between the divine Father and Mother aspects of being, as: spirit-matter; positive-negative; life-form; which when combined create the Divine Son or Christ within.

Humanity has distorted the divine nature of the sex energy through believing animalistic urges are true love impulses, through sexual magic and the abuse of tantric energy, and the stepping down of the divine nature into the animal realm. Sex has been used to satisfy the urges of the animalistic lower self at any cost, outside of normal spiritual rhythms.

In the world of material form that we reside within there are various aspects of the sex energy:

- The emanations from the very cells and tissues, and these are dependent on how coarse or refined the physical vehicle has been developed through the evolution of the soul. There are different emanations from a brutal animalistic person than from a spiritual person.

- Those vibrations coming from the animalistic-related aspects of the organism that create animal magnetism for the purpose of coming together to procreate and further the species. These will create forces of attraction and repulsion between people.

- Those emanations which are related to the harmonious patterns within the cells, and can allow the physical body to recognise the spiritual aspects of an interaction, and allows two people to feel the true harmonious relationship rather than simply bodily sexual attraction. Thus the vibration of knowing through the body whether it is divinely appropriate to have sexual links with someone, or whether doing so would create karmic disharmonious patterns and send soul parts of each person to alternate realities. These emanations are as yet little understood.

The sexual instinct also carries within its root the fear of separation and loneliness. Sex is then used in a lower form in order to avoid feeling separation and isolation in the material plane, and this has till now been needed to propagate the human species. The unthinking 'savage' has an approach to sex whereby it is guided by the rhythm of animal nature. The spiritually aligned person guides sexual expression through the mind and for the good of humanity. In between these two approaches are many points of view and sexual patterns. The sex energy is an aspect of the relation between the soul and the body, and is anchored in the mystic or divine marriage between the two. This involves a merger between the Mercury (Hermes) and Venus (Aphrodites) forces within the sacral chakra and the brain centres (creating the divine inner hermaphrodite).

Amongst the problems that have developed in the use of the sex energy on the planet is that the herd or animal instinct in sex has become distorted by various emotional patterns within humanity. This has created all sorts of distortions ranging from free love or promiscuity to rigidly restrictive or religious points of view where sex is considered sinful and to be denied. For example, the latter viewpoint was not the true teaching of Christ but became distorted within the Christian religion.

Humans have prostituted themselves and this has grossly distorted their sexual energies, creating perverted mental thoughtforms. This includes some of the mental illness today, as in depression and psychosis. Indeed the kidneys rule the sexual energy as well as the nerve energy. Diseases arising from kidney problems include dementia, depression and brain diseases. These principles can be illuminated when studied from the perspective of Chinese medicine. Many of the diseases today are related to the abuse of these sexual energies, even when they do not seem related, e.g. the gonorrhoea (sycotic) and the syphilitic miasms.

A cruel imposition has become placed on women to serve the sexual appetites of men, and much of society has become centred on this. Men have never really been monogamous over history. Instead they have sought the momentary pleasure of ejaculation, which confines their sexual powers to the animal plane. They have given themselves license to follow different rules of sexuality according to their culture and environment, thus depending on the area there can be polygamy, monogamy, promiscuity, prostitution, etc. and each culture either sees these as right or wrong. It has created red light districts on the planet with much vicious and violent energy being played out.

This promiscuity has led to an overpopulation of planet Earth, and souls have been forced into incarnation when they were not ready and not properly planned. It has also disrupted the economic life of the world. Indeed many millions of souls have been brought into the Earth through artificial and enforced birthing at a time when it was not intended for them to incarnate. This has created much of the economic and planetary distress, with the precipitation of war to reduce the excess proliferation of the race.

Disease results when humans do not regulate their sexual energy in line with the rhythms of nature. There are rhythms and cycles within the sexual energy, which is more obvious in the female through her menstrual cycles. At present males are not conscious of the rhythm within their sexual energy, and many of these cycles are in the mental plane. They will realise these with further evolution. Instead males disrupt the female cycles by having intercourse at times inappropriate to the common good. Birth control methods are used to allow such unregulated sex to occur. This distorts the sexual energy of both partners, especially the woman – to cause infertility problems.

The syphilitic miasm or disease began in Lemuria. It is a misconception to think that the earlier races of humanity were free from any type of contamination from sexual diseases. In Lemuria the emphasis was on developing the physical body, and sexuality focused heavily on the physical. Much misuse of sexuality occurred through mismatched mating, promiscuity and perversions. The sacral centre was the chakra undergoing collective evolution at the time. In the event the Lemurian race practically destroyed itself.

Over the aeons, burial of those who died of syphilis and similar such problems have caused the very soil of Earth to become permeated with syphilitic vibrations. This all needs to be cleared to return the Earth to its pristine nature. Part of this will be the increased use of cremation of the dead rather than burial, for fire allows the proper dissolution of vibrations left within the etheric body.

Cancer is the main disease stemming from abuse of power during Atlantis. Its causes are within the emotional and astral body, which was the body then under development. It was partly a reaction to the sexual excesses of Lemuria. The Atlanteans had to reduce and block the damaging effects of this excess by setting up energetic blocks in their own bodies, especially in those parts where the etheric body has a strong hold with less astral control, such as the reproductive organs and gastrointestinal tract. Cancer is mainly a disease of inhibition. The solar plexus was the main chakra then under development, and is a key focus for the cancer miasm. Whereas sex was the major area of sin in Lemuria, in Atlantis the major area of sin was theft, suppression and control. Theft included stealing parts of other souls (soul theft). This problem was widespread, and can be addressed for example through shamanic or energetic soul retrieval therapy.

The region where cancer develops has overactive but stagnant energy, with also suppression of the overall system and ineffectual cellular guidance by the mental and spiritual bodies. Cancer in the sacral centre has often been caused by well-intentioned suppression of the sexual energy by spiritual aspirants, many of whom during the post-

Atlantean epoch have had incarnations involving a celibate or monastic life. The soul in this case followed the line of least resistance to sexual temptation. During Atlantis sex was considered wicked and sinful, especially by religious leaders. Energy follows thought and magnetises physical changes, causing cancers and tumours.

In summary, when sexual desires are rampant and acted out, there arise diseases such as syphilis, genital inflammations and perverted sexual behaviour. When sexual desires are inhibited there arise cancers, lung congestion and tuberculosis (due to excessively flighty and romantic idealism in the soul). The temperament defines the disease.

Sexual evolution and the influence of the seventh ray

The solutions will not be found through religious, political or societal laws or regulations, but through a transformation of consciousness. The incoming ray for the new Aquarian age is the seventh ray of freedom and transformation (colour violet) and it works through the sacral centre of the planet, thus affecting everyone's sexual nature. It makes humanity look at its sexual patterns. The outgoing ray of the Piscean age is the sixth ray of devotional love, and there is somewhat of a clash between these two energies within humanity at present, illustrated by the conflict between religious dogma and the need for individual and group freedom. The seventh ray works through the sacral centre and the sixth ray through the solar plexus (with a link to the astral plane), thus desire and emotional conflict is caught up in world affairs today.

There are of course many spiritually aligned men and women who have resisted the temptations of the flesh and many have needed to be in ashrams or monastic environments away from the rest of the world. Also many people have avoided temptation out of fear of wrongdoing or for fear of sin. However the future will lead to union of the inner male and female energies again, but not in an androgynous or sexless way, but as a divine hermaphrodite, with balanced male and female energies. As the new impulses of untried and liberated sexual expression pour into the planet, it releases and brings to surface the old sexual patterns. Within weak human minds this shows as distorted sexual behaviour. Weak souls thus succumb to their lower nature. This is only a temporary surfacing of evil and prostitution of energy in material ways.

The coming of Christ is imminent, as a physical embodiment (but not necessarily as a single individual) and as collective Christ consciousness. This is not a promotion of any particular faith or religion, but relates to a world energy. Thus the influence of the seventh ray and the new age brings much collective co-operation, group effort, a desire for union with others as well as chaos and upheaval. These same impulses as felt by undeveloped bodies and souls leads to a desire for union, but in a lower based sexual way, both legitimate within marriage and illegitimate. Sexual unions therefore occur along intended evolutionary as well as unintended karmic lines. The new age stimulates both good and evil, with both material and spiritual aspirations activated. Overall the outcome is for higher development.

In a relationship there will be increasing union and harmony between the spiritual, mental, emotional and physical bodies of the partners. This becomes a divine marriage between the two people. Usually the present situation is a faint connection at only one body level, e.g. a marriage between the physical bodies of the two. Sometimes the emotional bodies are well connected, but rarely have the mental bodies been so. Or the physical body of one person may be interacting only with the emotional body of the other. In this case the emotionally connected person will probably have a physical cold, uninvolved and frigid experience, yet feel an emotional dependency or nurturing connection to the person in other ways. True union between two souls through all their vehicles must first be prepared through the inner development of the spirit within each person. This situation then provides the right conditions for the incarnation of souls, where the incoming soul can feel its God given powers properly anchored into the world. When the parents are essentially physically- and/or emotionally-based the child also becomes stuck in these aspects of its being.

Love and sex as terms are often used interchangeably, but the true meaning of love has become distorted. When used correctly they become one and the same energy, and allow expression of the law of attraction – and the expression of the relationship between God and human through that of man and woman. Spirit and matter thus meet together, in a productive fruitful union with the birth of the Christ.

The energies of the chakras below the diaphragm become raised to work through the chakras above it. This allows the emergence of beauty within form. The activation of the throat chakra for example allows the true expression of the power of the Word and increased creativity. Most people have been living from below their diaphragm and expressed their energies within the material realm. In future races the expression of energy will be from the heart, throat and head chakras. The head chakras bring in positively polarised masculine Father-God energy, and the brow centre brings in negatively polarised feminine Mother-God energy. Connected to these two are vortices of energy from the pineal and pituitary glands respectively. As the person spiritualises, the personality becomes purified and the body energy automatically elevates to become focused at the brow centre.

Thus sexual energy as union becomes manifest in three levels:

- In physical plane sex between man and woman for the procreation of new divine forms for incoming souls.

- In the union of lower energies with higher energies to bring creative work.

- In the union of the personality with the soul-spirit and through this the merger between the head/pineal with the brow/pituitary centres, to birth the Christed self.

The evolution of humanity over the passage of time has led to this great achievement on the Earth plane. More and more people on Earth are becoming creative in the fields of art, culture, politics, philosophy, science, etc. and the impact of this mental energy is changing the planet. However this creativity needs to overcome lower ego competitiveness in order to anchor collective sharing and transcendence of personal aims for transpersonal planetary evolution.

The three vibrations that have become active in sexual evolution and generally throughout human behaviour are from three of the planets. Thus Saturn is the first active influence and divides the many possibilities facing humanity so as to allow a choice as to that which anchors divine purpose. With this come feelings of discipline and discrimination. Later the influence of Mercury is felt, and with this is a pouring of light along spiritual and mental lines, and a sense of true interpretation of spiritual teachings. The initiate at this point seeks to unite the lower with the higher energies within the body and being, and fuse the personality with the soul. The third influence is from Venus, which governs intelligent love. Human group work now becomes important, with co-operation rather than competition. All this will influence the sexual and marital life on the planet.

As humans merge their subconscious mind with their conscious mind and learn of their threefold nature, and as education focuses more on spiritual matters, then men will have a change in attitude towards women and women will change their attitudes towards their life purpose and destiny.

The three generations of humans since the early part of this century have anchored each of these energies Saturn, Mercury and Venus in turn. Thus the generation with a childhood during 1920-1950 had particularly to deal with matters around abode, the right place to live and work (e.g. emigration to other lands, to set up families abroad) or issues around family responsibility. Saturn influenced their behaviour. The next generation, influenced by Mercury, had their childhood during 1950-1980 and was more particularly involved with bringing spirit to the Earth plane. The generations of children born between 1980-2010 have well equipped spiritual bodies to understand the life of the collective and have the Venusian influence. They will be able to successfully lead humanity out of the state it has got into. This is a fact and will happen.

There are always those at each great epoch and time of transformation who have incarnated with the ability to effect change. At each stage there is increased transpersonal positioning with a wider viewpoint. Future science and education will be based on guiding a person to understand their inner realms. Spiritual psychology will be part of the curriculum, including teaching children about their ray and vibrational makeup and an analysis of natal and other astrological horoscopes. There will thus be a sound basis to the development of mind and soul powers. Group effort, individual purity, ethos and alignment will be taught. Sexual relations will be based on intelligent guidance, appreciation and knowledge of the soul of one's partner. Of course the unthinking, lazy and dull-witted will still be found, but overall humanity will have evolved.

Marriage and relationship will be regarded through their effect on the group and collective good, not out of legal or religious binds but that which truly serves all. Men and women will thus know themselves as cells within a vital organism. Men will live less in the world of animalistic and unregulated desire and more in the mental and spiritual world with guidance over their lower sexual energies. The manner in which men express their sexual urges is presently abnormal, and as the throat and head chakras open there will be the realisation of what is right and of mutual benefit for both partners as well as for the collective.

Sex is an energy, which allows principles of life to bring together units of form to build a higher form. It involves the meeting of opposites into at-one-ment, to produce a third reality which bears witness to the other two. People will realise the truth of reincarnation and rebirth, and that each life is a re-capitulation of all that has happened/is happening/will happen; thus it will be felt that mistakes must not be allowed to happen in the sexual sphere. Humans will come to tread their path more carefully, and listen to their family and group collective obligations. Evil thought leads to karmic patterns as well as physical actions, thus placing more responsibility on the mental and spiritual life of everyone.

It is false to believe a spiritual person should be celibate or have no married life. This attitude has stemmed from a mistaken religious attitude towards women. Man is no better nor worse than woman. All are equal, indeed a human is divine and both male and female. It is not the men of the world who are to blame, for women have also been men in other lives as have men been women. There is no sphere of human life where a person cannot anchor their divine nature including sexual and marriage relations. If any of the energies of a person are frustrated and blocked, then that is damaging to spiritual awakening as well. Enforced celibacy is not a necessary part of spiritual evolution, and family life can evolve an initiate very well. Many ascended masters have had families and children. It is purifying to the initiate to bring their animal lower-based aspects to rhythmic discipline within a relationship, and to elevate their emotional bodies into sacrifice within the family. Many enforced attempts at celibacy have caused perversions and undue mental suffering for people on their path to enlightenment. Of course sometimes a person has to go through a period of celibacy to balance out the sexual excesses of a past life and to give the lower ego the time to readjust itself.

From seeing it as an animalistic furthering of the species or having a social/economic function parenthood will evolve into preparing and establishing a connection for souls from the spiritual world into the Earth world. Each parent has an individual column of light, called the antakharana, which integrates that person's spirit with the grid of incarnated personalities. Both parents donate part of their channels to form a united antakharana, which connects them to the incarnating soul. This is developed during the preconception stage.

The chakras and sexual energy

Mercury is particularly active in the sacral and throat chakras. The main chakra dealing with sexual energy is the sacral. It is very powerful and programmed to remain so until two-thirds of humanity have taken initiation enough to leave the cycle of rebirth. At this point the human race no longer needs the full procreative powers of the chakra to provide physical bodies for incarnating souls. It will then be governed intelligently through spirit and for the collective good rather than for personal animalistic lust filled sexual urges. The sacral chakra carries a blueprint for the entire gestation period of the physical body. This faculty extends to all aspects of material creation, including the creation of new ideas, organisations, projects, etc. Through this chakra the problem of duality can become resolved.

The sacral chakra was brought into functioning in Lemuria with the creation of the sexes (the male and female divisions of humanity). The physical manifestation of the sacral chakra are the gonads, which are identified as male or female (but not both male and female together within the system of duality). This segregation creates the urge to unite again with the other sex type. The spiritual disciple has to learn proper control of sexuality. Attempting to enforce abstinence and celibacy in the current life without development of balanced sexual control in former lives could present as repressed sexuality and perversions. In humans having lower levels of consciousness there is much psychic perception between themselves at the sacral chakra, with the solar plexus chakra regulating this psychic awareness. The chakras above the diaphragm are quiet. Their sex life is based on lower astral sentient feeling, thus having an ability to easily invite relationships based on emotional needs and fulfilment of their sexual appetite.

The sacral chakra must instead become transmuted and raised to function at the level of the throat centre, and then the person is able to use further creative forces to enter the spiritual realms. Upon higher development the routes for transfer of energy between the chakras are:

- The sacral chakra governs the mental elemental life and transfers to the throat chakra.

- The solar plexus chakra governs the astral elemental life and transfers to the heart chakra.

- The base chakra (with four petals) governs the physical elemental life and transfers to the crown chakra (an infinitely-petalled lotus flower).

As well as stimulating the higher chakras, the lower chakra must be properly controlled and transformed, otherwise problems such as fanaticism, unbalanced idealism, spaciness, impracticality, guru worship or spiritual ego states can result. The person is actually wandering around within the astral world of illusion rather then transcending this into higher spiritual worlds. Further examples arise if, for example, the heart energy transferred into the solar plexus – to cause personality power struggles. The person can actually become isolated as regards occult development, and use their energy to control others through the solar plexus. The emotional body is then out of alignment with the physical body as well as the spiritual and mental bodies. When energy in the sacral chakra is raised to the level of the solar plexus chakra there can arise various intestinal and digestive problems. This is due to completion of the problems stored in the sacral centre, but with release of latent buried problems in the solar plexus. This is of course ultimately required for true liberation from karma.

Much trouble is currently experienced by souls through a worldwide throat chakra opening within humanity. Excessive or premature activation can result in hyperthyroidism, which is an increasing problem. This can arise from the celibacy enforced on many people (through their inability to manifest the right relationship and thus deciding to avoid having any sexual relations). This blocks creative powers in the sacral chakra that would otherwise balance the opening of their throat chakra. Also much energy may be flowing into the throat chakra but the person is not making use of it for higher creativity. When the throat chakra is used properly it can raise the creative forces within the sacral chakra. The sex life becomes regulated and not wasted or spent to exhaustion through promiscuity. For this the personality must be properly integrated and this is a function of the brow chakra and the pituitary gland linked to it.

There is also the influence of the internal and latent fire forces or warmth energy. This warms the physical cells and the whole organism, and provides the basic energy for reproduction. If a person uses their will to activate fire forces prematurely then mental illness such as insanity, obsession and even death can result. There can be over-development of the sexual energy if the physical body is not pure enough to cope with the fire forces. The spinal pranic channel may well be blocked and clogged in this person and thus form a barrier to the kundalini energy, which can then travel retrograde or downwards, or even out of the spinal pranic tube altogether. This wreaks havoc on the etheric body and causes physical body damage.

Chapter 15

Mercury and Old Saturn in the skeletal anatomy

Mercury is structurally involved within the human shoulders, collarbones (clavicles), arms and hands. Deep esoteric significance lies in these relationships, and again involves the nature of the personality and its development. Creative impulses or formative principles underlie the skeleton. Such impulses are hidden behind the outward manifestation, and therefore grasped only by spiritual sight, and often a degree of faith and imagination. These are undervalued yet powerful tools for the spiritual seeker. The actual function of the skeleton will change as the human being anchors soul-spirit into the physical structure and this includes the awareness that the human has the ability to fly. The skeleton in fact balances the forces of gravity and Earth connection with those of weightlessness and buoyancy.

The clavicles

These are spiritually connected to the Keys of Solomon (an esoteric switch to receiving spiritual initiation). Note that they easily fracture. The name clavicle is derived from 'claviculus', Latin for a 'key', to which their S shape is similar (Fig. 15-1). When they are crossed, they look like the esoteric symbol of a swastika, which means life, expansion and movement. It is a bone of individuality. It is a long slender S-shaped bone with two curves. The medial one-third portion (nearer the middle of the body) is convex anteriorly, and the lateral one-third is concave anteriorly. At its medial end it forms a joint with the sternum (called the sternoclavicular joint). At its lateral aspect it forms a joint with the acromium part of the scapula. The clavicle transmits forces from the upper arm to the trunk, and if too severe a force (e.g. a fall on one's outstretched hand) it can cause a fracture of the bone.

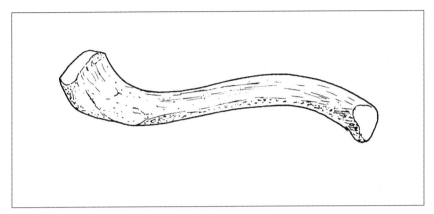

[Fig. 15.1] *Clavicle, showing slight sinusoidal shape and form.*

It is the first bone to ossify (laying down of mineral deposit in its structure) in the human embryo, during the fifth week. This indicates it is very ancient in its development on Earth. This is different from the usual scientific view that bones develop in response to their function and from the need to move muscles. A bone can develop before there is an apparent need for it, and form is not necessarily related to function. The ossification occurs in the centre (called primary centre) and is from a membranous matrix. The secondary centres (or epiphyses) of ossification develop in the periphery or outer parts of the clavicle and fuse around the age of twenty to twenty-five, preventing the bone from further growth. The other bones of the body that ossify from a membranous matrix are the flat bones of the skull vault and the bones of the face. All other bones of the skeleton develop out of cartilage, which reflects a later stage of Earth development.

Centres of ossification of a bone are sites of minor chakras. Minor chakras are found in many places in the physical, etheric, astral and mental bodies, e.g. behind the knees and in the medial elbows. Also, where a nutrient artery enters a bone there usually lies a site for a minor chakra.

The clavicle is fully developed only in the human and in some of the apes. In the animal kingdom it is generally small or even absent; instead the scapulae (shoulder blades) form the most important part of the shoulder girdle. Indeed in many of the animals, the clavicle does not articulate with any other bone at all, and is only embedded in muscle. Only animals that climb or grasp with their arms really have a clavicle, in the rest it has degenerated. The hands and arms are held away from the skeleton of the torso in humans, whereas it is bound closer to the torso of the typical animal skeleton. It is only in humans where the clavicles become fully developed so as to hold the upper arm humerus bone away from the vertebral column and sternum (breastbone). In animals the poor development of the clavicle ensures their arms and legs are similar in orientation and can both function for ambulating on all four limbs.

The clavicle allows a being to become upright, to escape from being Earth-bound and have a variety of arm movements. Note its relationship with the human skull bones which are also formed out of membrane in the embryo, and thus it has a link to the primary image from the Creator and the higher mind. These bones also relate to the individualisation that took place during the Moon chain prior to the formation of Earth. The Temple of Solomon relates to the greater human, Adam Kadmon, who is yet to be perfected. For this to manifest there is to be a second spinal cord, the re-emergence of certain extra glands, and a reduction in bone and tissue density in the human body over a future period.

Uprightness and the EL-shift

The upright stance of the human is however an expression of its personality rising above the linear third-dimensional programming of earthly space and time. This posture provides for the vertical alignment needed to anchor the ascension energy of spiritual realisation and experience the true source of the self in the starry heavens as a spiritual being incarnated on Earth. Underlying this is the principle of the EL-shift. 'EL' are the initial letters to the names of great spiritual beings called the Elohim and the Elders. The Elohim are vast creator-beings standing at the right hand of God. They are responsible for holding within their form, and indeed in becoming, the building block vibrations for creation. These are not the same as the crude atoms and subatomic particles theorised by material science, but are spiritual qualities such as Grace, Harmony, Peace, Charity, Hope, Trust and so on. These qualities are actually beings, which make up the substance of souls, spiritual beings and worlds.

Elders are related great beings responsible for travelling from one star and planetary system to another and programming them with the necessary blueprints for life support thereon. To use a principle from computer science, an initially uninhabited planet is hardware for the Elders to program the required software such as operating systems, BIOS (input-output systems) and the like. When programming the Earth, the Elders ensured they embedded the EL-shift, also written as L-shift. The letter 'L' has a horizontal and vertical configuration. The horizontal aspect encodes for consciousness bound by linear space and time, and is symbolised by the animal kingdom, which are bound to the nature forces of Earth. The vertical aspect encodes for the ability to ascend, or step out of linear space and time. It provides for the ability of the human soul in this planet to align to its spirit and leave the wheel of rebirth and reincarnation, unpinning from karma and duality on the planet.

The snake and the human pranic tube

The classic depiction of the horizontal positioning with respect to the EL-shift is the snake. This was the first creature that fell to Earth with its ego consciousness. In other words it was the first to incorporate its nervous system within a bony vault (the vertebral column) and thus limit its nervous system within the Earth's mineral kingdom. It symbolises the fall of humanity, as revealed in the story of Adam and Eve and their temptation in the Garden of Eden under the cunning persuasion of the snake. That the snake has lost its limbs and fallen to the ground and in many cases is practically blind and cold-blooded shows further its seemingly limited faculties on Earth.

However the snake (see p.84) also represents the ability to resurrect and redeem oneself, and contains powerful healing forces within its devic spirit or group-soul to this effect. More than any other animal species it has adapted to practically all terrain (from sea, river, tree-top, desert, frozen tundra and so on), to eating a wide variety of foodstuffs and to having several methods of killing and capturing prey. Many snakes even have thermal or heat sensors at the level of a third eye, which reveals ancient saturnine forces working through this creature. Mercury complements the snake forces and thus the homoeopathic snake remedies. It guides the transformative vibrations of a snake medicine into the physical and subtle bodies, to clear blocks in the spinal cord, vertebral column and underlying pranic or energy tube.

These properties are revealed by the symbol of the caduceus (see p.83). The two intertwined snakes running along the staff symbolise the sinusoidal metatronic waveforms running along the pranic spinal tube. These are electrical, magnetic and gravitational waves which travel from the alpha chakra (about 15-20 cm above the head) and the omega chakra (about 15-20 cm below the spinal base). They are multidimensional chakras not specifically linked to physical body regions. The alpha chakra carries the totality of one's spirit. The omega chakra carries the totality of all one's incarnations across the space-time grid (all the lives the soul has had in all planets, star systems and alternate realities). The pranic tube is a column of energy that conducts information and energy between these two centres and will thus carry all possible experiences and interactions of the soul.

For souls undergoing limitation during their incarnation the pranic tube will be highly distorted and have all sorts of etheric tears, holes and attached cords linking it karmically to other souls and entities. Thus the pranic tube and its physical counterpart, the spinal cord and vertebral column will not be fully 'owned' by the soul. The personality could be described as 'spineless', or 'without backbone', to any behavioural pattern where it does not have the consciousness and wherewithal to stand up for itself. Metatron, the King of the Archangels, is responsible for all light in manifestation and as yet unmanifest in the universes and creation. Of the three waves of Metatron, the magnetic wave carries spiritual qualities of will and power, and is aligned to the Father aspect of God as Trinity. The electrical wave of Metatron carries spiritual qualities of love and is aligned to the Mother aspect of God as trinity. The gravitational wave carries spiritual qualities of wisdom and mastery and is aligned to the Child or Christ aspect of God. These waves have deep practical significance, for repair and tonification of the pranic tube and clearing any blocks in the tube leading to proper activation of the waves will alter the whole energy makeup of the soul and its body vehicles.

Furthermore, when the magnetic wave is altered, this by necessity alters the magnetic field of the entire physical and subtle bodies and combined aura. This in turn changes the interaction between albeit the smaller magnetic field of the individual and that of the Earth, to the point that the planet actually adjusts its own magnetic field to synchronise the shifts. The same applies to changes in the individual electrical and gravitational waves. Thus fine-tuning of the pranic tube has profound consequences for the nature of Earth and the stability of the third-dimension. Such power to transform Earth reality is latent in the pranic tubes and spinal cords of most incarnated souls, until the necessary inner development has prepared them for responsible use of such power. Mercury is a key vibration required for smoothing this flow of metatronic energy along the pranic tube. Many spinal diseases can consequently be treated by homoeopathic application of Mercury.

The cosmic lemniscate form

There is a cosmic theme in the human skeleton that reveals itself as the lemniscate, or a figure of eight (8, also ∞). The unit of a vertebra and its two ribs shows the basic underlying shape throughout the skeleton. This can be seen as two enclosed cavities; at the back is the spinal canal between the vertebral body and its arches, and at the front is the space between the two ribs and sternum. The first space, the spinal canal, progressively enlarges as one ascends up the column into the head, whereas in the downward direction it progressively reduces in size to a dead end in the coccyx. It can be imagined the upward direction enlarges to infinity through the head into the heavens. On the other hand, the rib space gets smaller as one ascends to the first rib, and widens in the downward direction to the open floating ribs. This can be further imagined to continue downwards through the legs into the Earth. Adding the arms to these images allows a third aspect of human functioning, where the soul has a world of its own between the two contrasts of heaven and Earth.

The planets in their orbits around the Sun are seen to have strange wandering patterns when seen from the Earth, due to the 'illusionary' movements created by the Earth's travel. However this is not an illusion in the sense that these lemniscate like movements represent essential qualities of the planets. The lines of curvature of the arms and spinal/rib lemniscate can be viewed as reflecting the patterns of the planetary movements. Note the pictures of Mercury's travel above the Earth's western and eastern horizons over the course of the year (see p.44). The human lemniscate can also be re-drawn as a sitting Buddha, as well as re-drawn as a vertebral body. The human is indeed a cosmic being on Earth.

The skeleton and Saturn forces

The skeleton is the physical structure holding the energy of Saturn in the human body. Through the skeleton the soul has a structural basis for realising its destiny and life purpose on Earth. It provides the firmness of character required for the earthly ego or personality to house the spiritual self. Those higher spiritual beings called the mercurian Archai have been especially involved in incorporating the ancient warmth forces of Old Saturn into the skeleton, by way of the bone marrow in the core. Within the bone marrow are the formative forces and stem cells for producing the circulatory blood. The blood contains the warmth forces of the ego, not simply to warm the physical body but also provide the drive for life purpose. The skeleton thus contains and anchors the impulses from Saturn. These include the sum total of all the past life purposes. Thus all the past lives of the soul, each with their intentions, destinies and ambitions, are brought together through the vibration of Saturn. These memories are held within the skeleton of the soul's physical body and can be awakened in the present life consciousness as and when required. Such re-surfacing must occur for all unrequited and unfinished past life tasks to be resolved. If such past experiences were not brought to completion, then the clutter of open loops of energy would cause the material realm to suffer rifts in space and time. All that the soul wished to fulfil must be completed before it can ascend and properly merge back into the spiritual realm. This includes overcoming the failures of past lives.

Mercury is the planet responsible, through the Archai, for dredging up the past when it is required to do so. If too much of the past destinies are brought up to present consciousness then mental illness can result from a splintered personality structure unable to integrate the disparate signals. The personality would feel overwhelmed by the past-life memories of incomplete purposes, and lead to frustration, denial, guilt, depression and even schizophrenia. Indeed Mercury is linked to such states of mental illness and scattered personality states as a consequence of harsh aspects and links to Mercury, in the astrology chart. When past life patterns are resolved by the soul in the present life, Mercury can subsequently open up a new experience for the soul.

Mercury, as for all planets, varies its signal to the soul in accordance with the spiritual evolution of the soul. Younger immature souls tend to have much incomplete past life baggage that Mercury is duty bound to bring up usually in small quantities for resolution and completion. As the soul becomes more spiritually awake and advanced, there is not the same heavy clutter in the past soul records. Mercury then guides into the earthly life of the soul fresh new blueprints and destiny codes from the cosmos, functioning as messenger from the spiritual realm. At still more advanced levels of unfoldment, the soul functions at a collective level of consciousness, making decisions that have planetary and solar system consequences and on behalf of groups of beings. This level of responsibility authorises Mercury to guide into the soul's conscious awareness unfinished patterns within humanity as a whole. The soul can thus work on changing planetary memory for the collective, and enter (in a detached objective manner) the past lives of other souls' to assist their own journeys.

Further elaboration is required of the warmth forces carried by the human blood (see p.175). When the human soul is as yet functioning through a relatively unconscious state of lower personality, then the warmth forces of the blood conduct fiery zeal and destiny codes. These codes stream from Old Saturn under the behest of the ancient beings of Old Saturn as encapsulated by the Archai of Mercury. This blood warmth is literally infused with the warmth forces of the Old Saturn souls and the mercurian Archai are holding these ancient beings within this blood; they are also known as guardians at the threshold. When the personality sleeps and enters the dream state, then the blood coursing through the physical body is even more deeply connected to these guardians. The mercurian Archai similarly become more deeply bound to the destiny of Saturn. The human soul has thus given away its power and allowed its incarnated physical body to be controlled. This is because at the incarnated personality level the soul is unable to properly guide its individual destiny, which must instead become fixed by the guardians.

As the soul and personality structures merge closer then the soul can directly infuse its spiritual currents of self-determined destiny and cosmic purpose into the physical blood stream. The warmth of the blood of an enlightened soul in physical incarnation is subtly but very different qualitatively from that of the unenlightened soul-personality. The warmth of the former soul has been wrested free from the direct influence of the Old Saturn beings and mercurian Archai. This self-determined warmth provides the fiery energy for truly unconditional opening of the heart chakra, and reception into the physical heart of spiritual currents from the cosmos. It is only by radiating the warmth forces of spirit out of the heart, physically and spiritually, can the soul anchor its own individualised warmth into the bloodstream. In so doing the soul must face the guardian at the threshold, which represents the sum total of its shadow, its subconscious inner demons and issues of unrequited love (arising ultimately from its separation from the cosmos and spiritual realm).

Chapter 16

Mercury and dental anthropology

Dental anthropology is the study of the teeth from archaeological, fossil and human remains in order to deduce the biology of ancient communities, their course of evolution and to enable individual identification. Teeth have an anatomy and physiology distinct from the rest of the skeleton. Teeth are also unique in being particularly resistant to degradation over time even though they had also formed the most exposed part of the skeleton throughout the life of that individual. Dental remains can also be easily compared to the teeth of modern living humans.

The various techniques employed in dental anthropology include:

- Studies of teeth morphology (size, shape and variation).

- The development of teeth in relation to age of the individual.

- The occurrence and history of wear in the teeth, both on the individual and in the community as a whole.

- The relation between dental disease and the diet and environment of the community.

A study of the spiritual causes behind various derangements of the teeth is instructive not only for understanding Mercury, but also the syphilitic miasm. Much destruction of the teeth occurs in the third stage of syphilis (see p.153).

The resistance to degradation even after long term burial under the ground reveals the essential nature of the Mercury process in the context of the underworld (of Hades) as within the teeth. Mercury enables information to be preserved even though the material storing such information (the physical teeth) are sent to the subterranean and underworld realms of Earth. When buried underground, teeth become opened to the forces of this underworld, with its presence of various elementals with strong degradation, recycling and purifying properties. However the Mercury process within teeth enables them to resist such degradation, preserving a connection with the superconscious soul life of that individual and enabling such subconscious soul parts to return back to the whole being of soul-spirit at some later date.

There is some confusion within the science of dental anthropology due to the mistaken premise that humans are related to the primates (apes and monkeys). According to Darwinian evolution, the human is simply a more developed ape, and such primates can therefore be studied to understand many of the features of the human physiology. It is beyond the scope of this book to properly discuss the spiritual and esoteric principles behind evolution of the human species. However it can be said that the ape is more of a by-product or side branch of human evolution rather than the predecessor. In effect apes came from humans, and not the other way round.

Humans have two sets of dentition: the milk teeth (or deciduous dentition) that are partially formed at birth and erupt into the mouth during the next two years. These are gradually replaced by the adult teeth (or permanent dentition) which completely take over by the early twenties. In terms of the seven-year stages of soul-spiritual incarnation and development, the first seven years of life are characterised by the milk teeth and the adult teeth erupt properly during the seventh year. The completion of ego or character incarnation occurs at age twenty-one.

Each dentition or set of teeth (milk and adult sets) are divided in four quadrants, i.e. the upper left, upper right, lower left and lower right (Fig. 16-1). Within each quadrant of the adult teeth there are two incisor, one canine, two pre-molar and three molar teeth. Within each quadrant of the milk teeth there are two incisors, one canine and two milk molars. Thus there are thirty-two teeth in the adult set and twenty in the milk set.

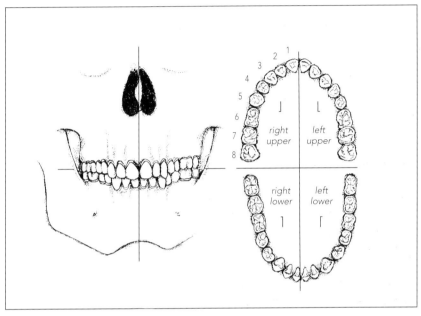

[Fig. 16.1] *Adult dentition with quadrants for nomenclature. There are thirty two teeth, divided into four quadrants. In the Zsigmondy system of denotion each quadrant is denoted thus: ⌋ upper right, ⌊ upper left, ⌉ lower right, ⌈ lower left. For example 4⌉ becomes the fourth upper right tooth, also known as the right upper first premolar.*

Structure of a tooth

Each tooth is divided into a crown and a root (Fig. 16-2). The crown is that part projecting into the mouth and is coated with enamel. The root is embedded into the jaw and is coated with a thin layer of cement. The whole tooth has a core tissue of dentine. The boundaries between the various tooth parts are called the enamel-dentine junction, the cement-dentine junction and the cement-enamel junction. Within the dentine there is the pulp chamber containing the soft tissue of the pulp. The floor of the pulp chamber opens through root canals into the jaw. The aspect of the crown which meets the opposite tooth crown is called the occlusal aspect and is a broad surface for the molars and premolars, but spatula-like for the incisors and canines.

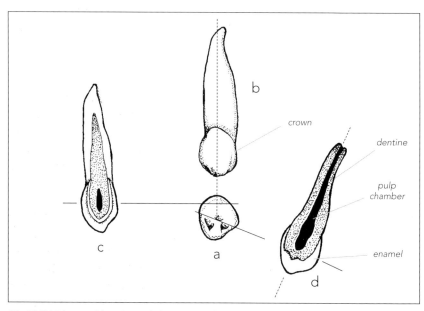

[Fig. 16.2] Adult upper right canine tooth showing internal structures. The crown is the portion projecting into the mouth, the root is embedded in the jaw. Dentine forms the core, and enamel the outer coating. The root is coated with a thin layer of cement. Inside the core is soft pulp with one or more root canals at its open floor. (a) Tooth occlusal aspect, (b) whole tooth, (c) tooth in transverse section and (d) transverse section through the central axis showing a root canal section.

The line of teeth along the jaw is called the dental arcade. The terms defining the various axis of tooth measurement are the crown length, crown breadth, crown height and root length. The tooth sockets within the jawbone have a lining of alveolar bone of a different consistency, and also a thin fibrous lining called the lamina dura.

The concept of species in spiritual dental anthropology

The scientific definition of species has relied on the uniqueness of certain features within the biological or material sphere. Thus a species is defined as a group of animals whose members resemble one another and under normal conditions only breed with each other. The reproductive and body structural boundaries defining them uniquely from other groups of animals is guided by the particular collection of genes they hold within their cells. They may of course vary amongst themselves and even vary markedly from other members of their species in other countries, but there remains a distinctive set of features, which distinguishes them from other species. The fossilised and modern remains of an animal can be identified to a particular species. Difficulties however remain in the variations that exist between males and females of many species; e.g. male gorillas are much larger than female gorillas, whereas in other ape or monkey species the genders may be similar in size. Therefore past records of extinct animals may need lengthy study to discover whether males and females had similar forms.

There is a difference in the blueprints defining the form in animals and humans. The group-soul of the animal species provides a common set of information to all animals within the species with respect to behaviour and characteristics of the animal. In short each animal receives the same program through the mercurial element of teeth. However the human is an individual and follows a personal biography in space and time, through a series of incarnations. The teeth of each human carry unique blueprints to do with the individual ego or character of that human. In most humans this set of information is tainted with the characteristic features of other humans, such as ancestors (including of course the parents), other members of the individual's soul group, and karmically linked aspects of other souls. In other words, each human is carrying informational baggage of other people within their body. Mercury conducts such information through the teeth.

When individuals becomes aligned to their soul-spirit, such baggage belonging to others is cleared from their consciousness, subconsciousness, and subtle and physical bodies. This instils a sense of freedom and mastery within the lower self. The vibration of the teeth also changes subtly, but profoundly – for the teeth are rather like a switch for new information to become conveyed into the bodies and genetic code. The person is effectively going through a 'teething process' of learning about themselves and their place in the world. Mercury conducts new and pristine codes direct from their soul-spirit into the physical body, locking these into the cellular genetic code. Notably tooth abscesses are common during this stage of re-alignment, and represent the clearing of etheric and physical debris of non-self from the teeth and the whole body.

Within the primates (apes) there is a high correlation between body size and tooth crown size. In other words, the larger the size of the ape's body, the larger is its teeth. This reflects the fact that memory and genetic programs in its physical body binds the animal. The animal must live in accordance with instinct, and this stems from the habit and past memory of its species. This memory is stored within the group-soul records of that animal species, which is the spiritual counterpart of the physical gene pool of that species.

However human souls are not so bound by instinct, past life memory, their ancestors nor by the general past of the human race. Each life that a human soul has is an opportunity to recreate their existence, to fashion a completely new and creative destiny within Earth and define an unexpected future for themselves and with respect to their contribution to the human race. Thus the human soul must not be restricted by any handicaps of the physical body, but may exercise the inner spiritual and mental resolve to overcome any such disability. Also the human baby incarnates with a potentially clean sheet with respect to its physical body, without the pre-programmed instincts and memories already awakened as in the animal; which is able to feed and survive with innate purpose already in its body. The strong correlation between the size of teeth in the ape and its body size is an indication of the clear reception of mercurial forces into the ape body. This provides an open channel for the spiritual realm to directly interface with the ape body and provide it with the information it needs to function on Earth. The human body is however seemingly blocked from receiving these mercurial codes so clearly, thus the human feels a sense of block and often frustration in the ability to physically perceive and follow their 'instincts'. The human makes mistakes in life that an animal would never make, simply because the animal feels always in harmony with the laws of nature and in resonance with the rest of Earth and the solar system. Humans have stepped out of harmony, but this gives them the capacity to feel individual, free-spirited and explorative. The mismatch between teeth size and body size provides for such a misalignment with the spiritual realm, and jams information from properly flowing from teeth to body and vice versa.

This is further revealed when comparing tooth crown size in different human populations. The largest average-sized crowns have been recorded in the Aborigines, and the smallest in Europeans and Asians. It is the indigenous native tribes of the world that have had the role of storing Earth memory and the history of the human race within their physical bodies and soul records. Thus the Aborigines, who are the oldest known remnant of ancient primitive peoples, have kept alive within their etheric bodies a rich tableau of Earth history. The size of their teeth directly reflects their ability to receive such information as memory and transmit it for storage within their bodies. Modern humans are however disconnected from Earth and human history. They are no longer able to directly recall their past lives, Earth energies or see into the subconscious realms. They have lost their intuitive awareness of reincarnation (which has remained nothing more than a vague recollection in some humans and a preposterous notion in many others). However, humans had to disconnect from their past in order to free themselves from ancestral and past life holds, and forgetting ultimately became a blessing rather than a curse.

The diameters of the teeth crowns has been measured and compared between fossil dentitions and modern dentition. Generally the (so called) primitive early stages of humanity, such as the Australopithecine (fossils found in East Africa and dating 4.4 to 2.5 million years ago) had larger canines and incisors and even much larger cheek (molars and premolars) teeth than later Homo species. Similarly, the teeth diameters has progressively reduced from early Homo habilis (about 2.2 to 1.6 million years ago in Africa) to Homo erectus (700 to 125 thousand years ago in Asia and Africa). There is further subsequent reduction in Homo sapiens archaic and Neanderthal (125 to 35 thousand years ago in Africa, Europe and Asia). The anatomically modern Homo sapiens (found since 90 thousand years ago with worldwide fossil records) have the smallest teeth of the series of human. The size reduction also applies to the milk teeth.

Furthermore a reduction in teeth crown diameter has been found during the evolution of the modern homo sapiens. A very rapid reduction in size occurred in early and late upper palaeolithic periods, more so in men than women. It correlated with a reduction in body size and strength. Postulated Darwinian-style theories to explain this include a change in diet, greater tool use and hunting tactics necessitating less powerful bodies for acquiring food. Thus the jawbones needed less strength to grind the softer and more cooked food. However such theories do not seem to satisfactorily explain the sudden reduction in teeth size, or the fact that some populations did have periodic enlargements in teeth and body size.

The giants

In the beginning every race and family of living species was androgynous, then at later times hermaphrodite and one-eyed. It is only later that two physical eyes developed in both animals and humans. In ancient humanity there are many references to giants, titans and cyclops. These actually existed, and belonged to the third root race (Lemurian) and fourth root race (Atlantean). They had superhuman physical power, and were able to defend themselves against the dinosaurs and other gigantic monsters yet to be discovered. It is only in this current fifth root race that humanity has developed a symmetry and relative perfection of form. Early fourth root races included beings with three eyes. This is because spiritual and psychic involution (or descent into matter) occurs in parallel with physical evolution (ascent of matter into spirit). Thus the inner senses have atrophied as the external sense have developed.

In Lemuria, there were initially androgynous (sexless) and then hermaphrodite forms, i.e. both male and female. Some of these early beings also had four arms and two faces, facing to the front and the back. The three eyes allowed them to see to their front and also from the back of their head. As humans descended further into matter, the spiritual third eye degenerated and humans lost their spiritual sight.

In later Atlantis, the inner spiritual vision was reactivated but by artificial means. During this process the pineal gland and third eye degenerated even further. The two faces also degenerated into one face, and there was only one eye, drawn deeper into the head so as to become hidden in the hair. Nowadays in meditation this buried pineal eye-like structure can be activated. During the petrification of the pineal gland in Atlantis, mineral deposits were placed within the pineal, which reveals the activity of the ego working deeper into the mineral kingdom to form a skeleton as an outer image of itself. The pineal is thus also called the Eye of Shiva, and carried the death forces of this deity. Due to its past connection to an eye at the back of the head (as a second face) the pineal gland presently can guide and connect to the alta major chakra, which is linked to the medulla oblongata at the brainstem (the back of the upper neck). In this way the pineal can regulate and inhibit when necessary the autonomic body control centres in the medulla (of sexuality, breathing and circulation).

It can be surmised that there is a deficiency in the fossil records (although various records have been withheld from public knowledge as they would show astonishing stages within human evolution, including the existence of giants). The early androgynous and sexless races of humanity in early Lemuria were indeed giants compared to the modern size of humans. The impulses of Mercury, as well as Venus and Mars, were needed to instil the required blueprint for sexual and gender differentiation within the human form. The blueprint for maleness came out of the cosmos from a different source than that for femaleness. Later the human size also required reduction and various physical faculties (such as supernormal senses, great speed and strength) were lost to provide for the relatively smaller and weaker present human form.

However, this has provided the impetus for the human soul to develop the faculties of the mind and spirit to overcome physical weakness. The teeth were altered so those blueprints (including genetic) as channelled through Mercury were more and more limited to those from the individual's own subtle bodies and soul-spirit. Thus the physical form had to rely less and less on support, by way of information, from the ancestors, relationships and guides of the soul. The soul had to become more self-sufficient and self-reliant. This is evident in the weakness and early decay of the teeth of modern humans, for the hardening and mineralising forces of the soul-spirit are poorly manifest in the physical body through a poor incarnation into the present life. The rapid reduction of teeth size during the recent evolutionary history of humanity occurred at such a time of separation of humanity from its etheric roots, and with it a gradual weakening of the strength and support humans could feel from their ancestors, the gods and spirit guides. Indeed early humans could actually feel the energy of their ancestors coursing through their blood and muscles, and felt themselves to be a living part of this rich ancestry – but this is of course no longer the case.

Odontoglyphics

This is the speciality within dental anthropology which studies the very specific pattern of grooves, furrows and mounds on the occlusal surfaces (biting surface of the crowns) of the teeth. There is a distinctive pattern analogous to the fingerprints, which can be used for identification of the individual. Concordance has been found in such patterns in the teeth of identical twins. There is suggestion therefore of a very high level of genetic inheritability in the pattern on the teeth crowns. Furthermore it can be stated that the patterns on the teeth crown are a visible and firm deposition of the specific blueprints of the self, the ego or individuality with respect to its particular characteristics in the present incarnation. In other words, the shape, size and pattern on the surfaces of the crowns represent the unique identity of the individual. They are rather like a switch for and an externalised marker for the individual's genetic code. By that is meant not the material set of genes on the cellular chromosomes but the morphogenetic field of information concerning the individual features and stored in the spiritual realm (and brought into holographic manifestation as the genetic code). The chromosomes are but string-like traces of energy with the imprint of information concerning the individual. In the future, humans will come to respect the role the teeth play in shaping the growth and development of the rest of their physical bodies as well as subtle body functioning (emotional, mental and spiritual bodies) and to honour the sanctity of the teething process in children. Mercurial information becomes blocked if this teething process is interrupted.

Malocclusion of teeth

Occlusion is the way in which the teeth fit together within the jaw. Thus the cusps and grooves within the lower cheek (molar and premolar) teeth fit exactly within the shapes of the upper cheek teeth when the mouth is closed. The edges of the upper incisor teeth overlap at the anterior edge of the lower incisors and the canines make a partial opposition to each other. For perfect occlusion the dentition must be completely perfect, regular and symmetrically arranged – although very few people actually have this (Fig. 16-3).

Unless it is marked, malocclusion tends not to adversely affect normal biting and grinding actions. Significant malocclusion can occur in abnormalities of teeth development, various genetic abnormalities, congenital absence of some teeth or extra teeth, impacted teeth and retention of milk teeth into the adult stage. These can all cause crowding of the teeth, abnormally excessive spacing, irregularity of shape and abnormal under or over-biting. The general subtle energy abnormality is the inability of the lower bodies to receive the blueprints from the higher bodies. The number three typically defines many of the relationships between spiritual and material. Thus there is the lower triad of bodies as physical/etheric, emotional and lower mental – which interface with the upper triad of astral, upper mental and spiritual bodies. Mercury guides the blueprints communicated between the two

HOMOEOPATHY OF THE SOLAR SYSTEM: MERCURY

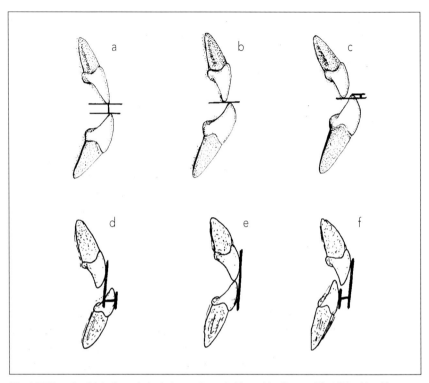

[Fig. 16.3] Normal and defective occlusion in the anterior teeth: (a) openbite, (b) normal bite, (c) overbite, (d) underjet, (e) normal edge to edge bite, (f) overjet.

spheres of the soul's activity. Disorders arising in the lower triad will distort the clear reception and expression of energy from the upper triad. The spiritual principle 'as above, so below' becomes upset, creating a tainted expression of the spirit in the material realm. Malocclusion is a clear sign of such a disturbance (usually genetic, ancestral and early childhood developmental) of the lower bodies. Such teeth derangement is typical of the syphilitic miasm.

Diastema
This describes abnormal gaps between teeth (Greek for intervals) and is more common in the upper teeth than the lower. Only some individuals have gaps between all the upper front teeth, commonly

there is only a single gap between the two first incisor teeth. The spiritual significance of a diastema is also a gap or interval but in the transmission of spiritual blueprints by Mercury. It is due to a lost life or experience between incarnations. The soul suffers a period in limbo with unresolved and stuck experiences between material incarnations, invariably in the lower astral realm and underworld regions (of Hades or hell). Examples include suicidal victims, drug overdose deaths, obsessive-compulsive states within the mental body and becoming trapped within the dense electromagnetic smog of the current digital age, when the soul finds it difficult to transcend the lower astral plane and enter the higher mental and spiritual realms after physical body death. In all these situations the soul is unable to receive new information through Mercury from the spiritual realm, but must first disengage from the problem. It is rather like being stuck in no man's land.

Irregular rotation and winging of teeth

Very slight twisting or rotation of the anterior (incisors and canines) is very common, to the extent that most dentists would treat it as practically normal. Excessive rotation can show as winging of teeth (Fig. 16-4) and this can be in one tooth in relation to its neighbour (unilateral winging) or both teeth in relation to each other (double winging). The rotation is towards the anterior or open mouth face. When posterior rotation occurs, towards the throat region, then it is termed counter-winging.

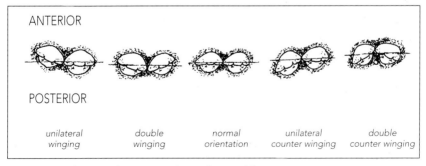

[Fig. 16.4] Upper first incisors showing various degrees of winging defects.

Winging is a sign of an abnormality of the forces of flight within the astral body and existence of stuck soul parts in the spiritual and/or subconscious realms. Mercury is noted to have three sets of wings as follows:

- First set: his helmet wings enable proper flight within the spiritual realm and thus proper communication with the cosmos of stars. These wings resonate with the sphenoid bone within the human skull, which is actually shaped like a winged structure when isolated at its suture junctions from the other skull bones. Note the sphenoid bone is also remarkably similar in appearance to the sacro-iliac or pelvic bones, revealing the need for aerodynamic balance between the head and base poles for graceful flying motion (Fig. 16-5).

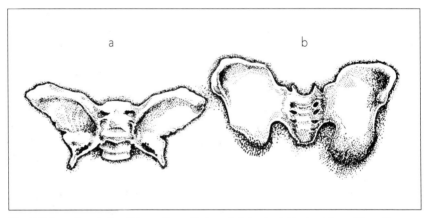

[Fig. 16.5] Comparison of sphenoid bone with sacroiliac bones (anterior views): (a) sphenoid bone, (b) sacroiliac bones.

- Second set: the chest wings spanning out of the pectoral region. These are the wings of the body proper, enabling flight within the third-dimension or manifest Earth realm. They are related to the form and function of the scapulae or shoulder blades. When both are placed beside each other note their resemblance to wings (Fig 16-6).

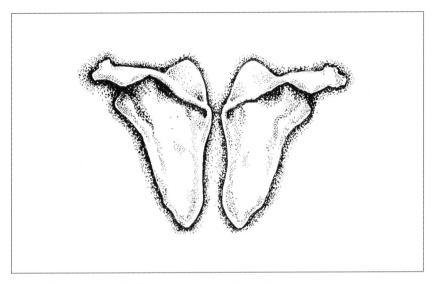

[Fig. 16.6] Both scapulae (shoulder-blades) posterior view and placed beside each other.

- Third set: the foot wings on Mercury's sandals are an expression of his ability to fly within the underworld of Hades, or the subconscious and subterranean realms of Earth. They resonate with the human astral body's ability to move the physical body with grace and ease within the material plane. When the astral body is poorly incarnated into the physical-etheric body then the latter feels slow, sluggish and too earthbound. The arch of the human foot is an expression of the buoyancy brought to the physical skeleton by this flighty astral body. The arch provides for etheric energy to not only descend but also ascend the legs from the Earth's grid of energy (which includes the electromagnetic Earth acupuncture meridians and subtle leyline grids). When humans loses their sense of buoyancy and spirit, the feet are liable to lose their arch and become flat (a sign of depression and weariness). Many forms of arthritis also cause loss of the foot arch. This goes especially for mutilating diseases with neuropathic joints where paralysis of sensory nerve function causes loss of joint position sense and pain perception. Any subsequent minor injury (such as stepping on a pin) is left unnoticed by the person, leading to joint destruction, sometimes from infection but more usually from chronic wear. Prime examples are syphilitic joints (also called Charcot-Marie-Tooth arthritis), psoriatic arthropathy and rheumatoid arthritis.

When the expression of the astral body is blocked at the sphenoid bone of the skull or the arch of the feet, with attendant cramping of the astral body elsewhere (invariably causing pain such as further arthritis and neuralgia) then winging of the teeth is more likely to occur. It is a sign of cramp of the astral body.

Impacted teeth
These are teeth that fail to erupt out of the jaw, and therefore do not properly meet the tooth at the opposite jaw. The tooth may attempt to erupt but do so in a distorted manner, such as sideways into the neighbouring tooth. The most common tooth to impact is the third molar, followed by the upper canine.

Impaction is a sign that blueprints as normally guided by Mercury are stuck and trapped in the realm from which they originate. For example stuck elements of the human soul, in the underworlds of Hades or the subconscious, or the lower astral plane, often lead to the rest of the soul being unable to proceed gracefully into the next incarnation. However if the soul were to newly re-incarnate then a part is missing in a unresolved situation in that other realm. This is an indication for using shamanic techniques of soul retrieval or soul rescue to guide that missing aspect of the soul back into its proper whole place. The incarnated personality subsequently feels more centred, grounded and balanced again.

However impaction is also a sign of a veil in consciousness and energy preventing this proper re-integration. It is a common scenario when a child fails to shed the morphogenetic blueprints of its parents and other ancestors during the first seven years of its life, thus retaining such holding patterns in its physical and etheric body, perhaps for the rest of its incarnation. This would occur if fevers are suppressed through anti-pyretics and infections not properly cleared by the child's own immune system due to the distorting effect of antibiotics. This restricts the blueprints governing the child's own physical and etheric body from descending into these bodies from the spiritual realm. The child does not then feel sufficiently free from the parents during the second seven-year period of age eight to fourteen and during the teenage period age fourteen to twenty-one. This can create various developmental disorders of the soul, including depression, co-dependency and confusion of life-purpose. This block to receiving its proper blueprints into the physical-etheric bodies is indicated by the distorted or ineffectual eruption of the adult teeth and abnormal retention of the milk teeth.

Congenitally absent teeth
This is a common finding in human dentition and is the lack of certain teeth to form at all (also called agenesis). It can be difficult to discern this diagnosis from impaction of that tooth, or loss of the tooth through injury or disease, i.e. situations where the tooth had actually formed. The most common tooth to miss out on formation is the third molar, and up to one-third of some populations studied have been found to have agenesis of this tooth. Agenesis is strongly associated with most of the other abnormalities of the teeth as discussed in this section.

The spiritual meaning behind this is the absence of any attempt to receive certain required blueprints from the spiritual realm into the physical–etheric body. Whereas impacted teeth revealed a stuck aspect of the soul, but which was attempting to re-integrate with the rest of the incarnation, in agenesis there is no effort made by the soul to retrieve its missing aspect. The soul has decided to learn its lesson with respect to that particular experience in some other life, which is usually future oriented or parallel in existence. In other words there is an apathy of the mercurial and other guiding forces from the soul-spirit to form a proper vehicle to express the soul's intent in the present incarnation (with respect to a certain lesson or set of lessons). Usually the soul has not resolved a death experience in some former past life, thus leaving an experience incomplete in that alternate reality – which is subsequently unable to re-integrate with the rest of the soul for some considerable time.

Supernumerary teeth
These are extra teeth (also called polygenesis) and are also usually of abnormal appearance. They may appear tucked in behind the normal teeth or to the side, lying between the normal teeth. Sometimes they do not erupt out of the jaw and are found on x-ray investigation.

The spiritual message behind supernumerary teeth is the abnormal retention of spiritual body blueprints from other lives of the soul. Invariably this means unresolved and unfinished karma and tasks left over from these other lives. This is of course common in general for human souls, but in this case there is a flood of information from these other realities of the soul without the physical body being able to cope with the increased workload placed upon it. Often there is also too much information streaming into the soul from ancestors connected to the genetic inheritance of the present incarnation.

Retention of milk teeth
Sometimes a milk teeth remains in the dentition, often with failure of eruption of its corresponding adult tooth. It is a sign of failure to properly activate the warmth forces of the child's ego consciousness during the first seven-year period of childhood. Hence its sense of self has a relatively poor grasp of its physical body. There was insufficient clearing from the physical-etheric bodies by the child of the blueprints carried from the parents and rest of the ancestors. Thus holding patterns from these ancestors remain in the child's body, possibly for the rest of its life – disabling it from following its true destiny with full possession of its physical vehicle. The milk tooth represents this retained information from the parents and ancestors. Ideally the situation should resolve by strengthening the child's character forces sufficiently to enable it to shed this tooth by itself, thereby exercising its ego life for the future.

Sequence and timing of dental growth

The usual length of gestation of the human embryo within the womb during pregnancy is thirty-eight weeks. Most babies are born somewhere between thirty-four and forty-two weeks. The onset of teeth formation starts around fourteen to sixteen weeks of gestation, these being the deciduous or milk teeth. The blueprints brought through Mercury for providing these teeth are constrained by the parental and other ancestral patterns. This is often a severe delimitation for the incarnating soul, for it must first clear blocks carried within its ancestors before embarking on its life purpose proper. This process is made much easier by the appropriate meditative and healing techniques to assist the mother and embryo to shed genetic patterns before the actual birth. These techniques are beyond the scope of this book and will be found in my 'Manual of Spiritual Healing'.

Of the permanent adult teeth, only one of the molars develops before birth, and remains within the jaw to erupt later. The rest of the permanent dentition begins to develop during the first three years of life, and the tooth crowns become complete around seven years of age. It is not until the early twenties of age that the tooth roots of these permanent teeth become complete. All the permanent teeth develop underneath the equivalent erupted milk teeth, except for the molars, which are without such a correspondence. As the roots of the milk teeth become absorbed the adult set of teeth can erupt.

There are thus three stages of the dentition:

- Period of milk teeth, generally up to age seven years. This period represents the submergence of the child's physical body within the parental and ancestral energy; its soul having a dim vegetative consciousness as yet largely hovering above its physical body.

- Period of mixed teeth, when the permanent adult molars erupt at the distal (far) end of the tooth row and the milk incisors are replaced by the adult incisors. This process occurs in sequence for the teeth during roughly the period five to twenty-one years. This period represents the overcoming of the parental and ancestral influences by the soul of the child, until it can become initiated into the world as a fully-fledged ego or individuality at the age of twenty-one years.

- Period of permanent adult teeth, when all the milk teeth have been replaced. This should have occurred by the early twenties and indicates that its ancestors no longer bind the soul.

Dental enamel

Enamel itself is a mineral deposit without cells, but is formed by a membrane of cells called ameloblasts. Initially there is a secretion of a matrix composed of one-third organic tissue (proteins and organic fibres) and two-thirds minerals. Through a special process of cell movement and matrix secretion there arises a network of pits in a hexagonal pattern. After the entire matrix has been laid down, the organic component is re-absorbed and the mineral fraction grows, but the network of pits is retained. These pits appear as regular lines or channels within the enamel and are called prisms or rods (Fig. 16-7). The prisms are packed in vertical rows that are layered next to each other.

The prismatic layered channels interconnect with channels running through the underlying dentine and thereby with the blood vessels supplying the root and gum area. There is constant flow of nutrient along these channels to the extent that enamel undergoes continuous regeneration. It is a living tissue albeit the hardest substance in the body. Indeed crowning and filling teeth with inert dead substance such as metal alloy or porcelain will block this nutrient flow to cause further deterioration of adjacent tooth substance. It tends to also cause deterioration in the health of internal body organs and tissues. The teeth provide a morphological reflex map of the whole body. Each tooth resonates with a particular region and tissue of the rest of the organism, rather like the map of the whole body within the feet in reflexology or within the ear Chinese acupuncture. The technique of

MERCURY AND DENTAL ANTHROPOLOGY

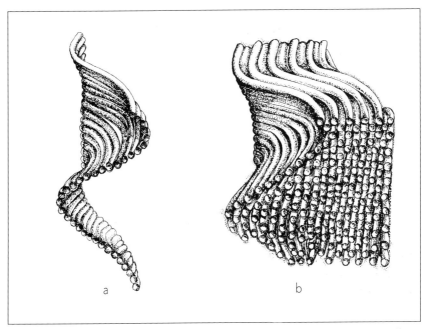

[Fig. 16.7] *Course of prisms within tooth enamel, showing sinusoidal arrangement: (a) single prism, (b) collection of prisms.*

electrodermal acupuncture involves measuring the skin surface resistance with an ohmmeter to find abnormal levels of electrical activity in relation to the acupuncture meridians and acupoints. Many investigators have observed resonance between these measurements and problems in particular teeth. The writer has integrated this information with further clinical and meditative study into the table of teeth-body correspondences (Fig. 16-8).

The special significance of the prismatic structure of enamel is it enables blueprint information to flow between the various space-time co-ordinates within which the soul resides. In other words, information can flow along the threads of consciousness that integrate the multiple incarnations and experiences of the soul into the experiences of one spiritual self. The prisms connect the 'bits' making up the self-identity together. Without the organised prisms, the self can appear fragmented

HOMOEOPATHY OF THE SOLAR SYSTEM: MERCURY

UPPER JAW

	8	7	6	5	4	3	2	1	1	2	3	4	5	6	7	8
nervous system & thinking faculty	lower spinal cortico-spinal tract	middle and upper spinal cortico-spinal tract	brain stem & cerebellum	limbic area, speech	temporal lobe, speech	parietal lobe, somato-sensory cortex	pre-frontal lobe, somato-sensory cortex	frontal lobe	frontal lobe	pre-frontal lobe, somato-sensory cortex	parietal lobe, somato-sensory cortex	temporal lobe, speech	limbic area, speech	brain stem & cerebellum	middle and upper spinal cortico-spinal tract	lower spinal cortico-spinal tract
sensory organs	6th csf ventricle	internal ear, hearing sense	5th csf ventricle	nose, smell sense	tongue, taste sense	3rd csf ventricle	lateral csf ventricles			lateral csf ventricles	3rd csf ventricle	tongue, taste sense	nose, smell sense	5th csf ventricle	internal ear, hearing sense	6th csf ventricle
endocrine system and chakra	psychic faculty, ESP	para-thyroids, R side	thyroid, R lobe	pancreas	thymus	adrenals R side, posterior pituitary	crown chakra, pineal gland	eyes and visual sense	eyes and visual sense	crown chakra, pineal gland	adrenals L side, posterior pituitary	thymus	pancreas	thyroid L lobe	para-thyroids L side	pituitary anterior lobe, esp growth axis
spinal cord and vertebrae	pituitary anterior lobe, esp. growth axis	lumbar L3-L5	lumbar L1-L3	thoracic T7-T12	thoracic T3-T7	thoracic T1-T2 Cervical C6-C7	cervical C3-C5	cervical C1-C2	cervical C1-C2	cervical C3-C5	thoracic T1-T2 Cervical C6-C7	thoracic T3-T7	thoracic T7-T12	lumbar L1-L3	lumbar L3-L5	sacral S1-S5
sinuses/air and csf systems	sacral S1-S5	parasympathetic nervous system, especially vagus nerve	bronchioles R lung	maxillary sinus, ethmoidal cells, major bronchi R lung	frontal sinus, larynx	sympathetic nervous system and spinal ganglia	sphenoidal sinus, frontal sinus, pharynx, trachea airway			sphenoidal sinus, frontal sinus, pharynx, trachea airway	frontal sinus, larynx	maxillary sinus, ethmoidal cells, major bronchi L lung	bronchioles L lung	parasympathetic nervous system especially vagus nerve	balance within both nerve systems	
muscular and skeletal systems	balance within both nerve systems	alveoli and connective tissue of lungs	R upper arm, humerus	R clavicle, scapula	R shoulder joint	facial bones, upper rib cage	skull: scalp and basal bones, upper rib cage	R kidney & urinary bladder, anus, rectum	L kidney & urinary bladder, anus, rectum	skull: scalp and basal bones, upper rib cage	facial bones, upper rib cage	L shoulder joint	L clavicle, scapula	L upper arm, humerus	alveoli and connective tissue of lungs	
organs	alveoli and connective tissue of lungs	R hand, wrist, elbow	small intestine and stomach, R side	R colon	R colon, R liver lobe, gb, R side of heart	R liver lobe and gb, R side of heart	L liver lobe, L biliary ducts, gb			L liver lobe, L biliary ducts, gb	heart (especially L side) and circulatory system	L colon	Small intestine and stomach, L side	L hand, wrist, elbow	duodenum, L side. Gut digestive activity	
	R hand, fingers	duodenum, R side. Gut digestive activity														
	3rd molar	2nd molar	1st molar	2nd premolar	1st premolar	canine	2nd incisor	1st incisor	1st incisor	2nd incisor	canine	1st premolar	2nd premolar	1st molar	2nd molar	3rd molar
Right	8|	7|	6|	5|	4|	3|	2|	1|	1|	2|	3|	4|	5|	6|	7|	8| L

MERCURY AND DENTAL ANTHROPOLOGY

LOWER JAW

Right	8|	7|	6|	5|	4|	3|	2|	1|	|1	|2	|3	|4	|5	|6	|7	|8	L
	3rd molar	2nd molar	1st molar	2nd premolar	1st premolar	canine	2nd incisor	1st incisor	1st incisor	2nd incisor	canine	1st premolar	2nd premolar	1st molar	2nd molar	3rd molar	
organs	duodenum, small intestine R side	small intestine, R stomach, R ascending colon		R side tranverse colon	R colon, R liver lobe, gb, uterus	R liver lobe, uterus	lower oesophagus, prostate, anus, rectum, urinary bladder, R kidney	lower oesophagus, prostate, anus, rectum, urinary bladder, R kidney	lower oesophagus, prostate, anus, rectum, urinary bladder, L kidney	lower oesophagus, prostate, anus, rectum, urinary bladder, L kidney	jejunum, biliary ducts L liver lobe, stomach, spleen, heart (esp. inter-ventricular wall uterus	L colon transverse, small intestine, L heart	L colon transverse, small intestine, L heart	colon (descending, sigmoid), L heart, aorta		terminal ileum (small intestine)	
muscular and skeletal systems	R foot distal phalanges	proximal R foot, ankle joints	R ankle joint	R knee joint	R knee joint, femur	sacro-iliac joint, lower rib cage	sacro-iliac joint, pelvis, lower rib cage	pelvic floor, R pelvic & hip joint, lower ribs	pelvic floor, L pelvic & hip joint, lower ribs	sacro-iliac joint, pelvis, lower rib cage	sacro-iliac joint, lower rib cage	L knee joint, femur	L knee joint	L ankle joint	proximal L foot, ankle joints	L foot distal phalanges	
sinuses/air and csf systems	alveoli and connective tissue R lung		terminal bronch-ioles R side	maxillary sinus, ethmoid, major bronchi R side	maxillary sinus, ethmoid, major bronchi R side	frontal sinus, larynx	sphenoid, pharynx, trachea airway	sphenoid, frontal sinus, pharynx, trachea airway	sphenoid, frontal sinus, pharynx, trachea airway	frontal sinus, larynx	maxillary sinus, ethmoid, major bronchi L side	maxillary sinus, ethmoid, major bronchi L side	terminal bronch-ioles L side		alveoli and connective tissue L lung	
spinal cord and vertebrae	sacral S1-S5	lumbar L3-L5	lumbar L1-L2	thoracic T7-T12	thoracic T3-T7	thoracic T1-T2 Cervical C6-C7	cervical C3-C5	cervical C1-C2	cervical C1-C2	cervical C3-C5	thoracic T1-T2 Cervical C6-C7	thoracic T3-T17	thoracic T7-T12	lumbar L1-L2	lumbar L3-L5	sacral S1-S5	
endocrine system and chakra	integration between cns especially limbic system with endocrine; R gonads (2nd molar)		R gonads	spleen, pancreas R side	spleen, pancreas	adrenal glands R side	adrenal glands R side		adrenal glands L side	adrenal glands L side		spleen, pancreas L side	spleen, pancreas	L gonads		integration between cns especially limbic system with endocrine; L gonads (2nd molar)	
sensory system	earth elemental and nature awareness			subconscious awareness	subconscious awareness	base chakra grounding	Metabolic eye (in the liver) and unconscious realm	Metabolic eye (in the liver) and unconscious realm	metabolic eye (in the liver) and unconscious realm		base chakra grounding	subconscious awareness			earth elemental and nature awareness	
nervous system & thinking faculty	spinal cord and cns integration		brain stem & cerebellum	limbic area, speech, temporal lobe	parietal lobe R side	somato-sensory area, esp. to legs	pre-frontal cortex	frontal lobe, corpus callosum	frontal lobe, corpus callosum	pre-frontal cortex	somato-sensory area, esp. to legs	parietal lobe L side	limbic area, speech, temporal lobe	brain-stem & cerebellum		spinal cord and cns integration	

[Fig. 16.8] Table of teeth/body correspondences. Explanation of abbreviations: cerebrospinal fluid (csf), gallbladder (gb), right sided (R), left sided (L).

237

and cause disorientation and alienation of personality incarnations within the soul. Again a mercurial quality is found in the prism and its picture of pathology. Notably each prism undulates from side to side in a sinusoidal manner like a waveform. It is similar to the waveform of the syphilitic bacteria, as well as the serpents of Mercury's caduceus.

Normally the surface of a tooth crown is smooth, white and mildly translucent. The defects that can arise are:

Hypoplasia of enamel
Where there is a deficiency of enamel thickness, this disrupts the normal contour of the crown surface. It is due to abnormal enamel matrix secretion during the growth phase of the teeth. It occurs in the unerupted adult teeth of children with rickets, scurvy, measles and smallpox. It has also been found in the milk teeth of children who suffered birth trauma, malnutrition, chronic allergies, congenital defects, anaemia, diabetes or syphilis. In all these conditions in various forms the ego consciousness or self-identity of the child is not able to assert itself within the physical incarnation, resulting in a weak activity of formation and differentiation of physical tissues. This especially occurs in the skeleton, teeth and nervous systems as key centres of activity of the ego consciousness.

Opacities and hypocalcifications
These are opaque white patches in the normally translucent enamel and are due to poorly mineralised areas under the surface, which reflect more light to the observer. It is another sign of a poor ego incarnation, with inability to take hold properly of the calcium metabolism.

Dental fluorosis and staining of teeth
This can occur from excess absorption of fluoride in drinking water. This causes opacities that stain brown through taking up pigments in food or from degenerated plaque. It is another sign of a weak ego incarnation, but this time with an inability to overcome the fluoride element within teeth through inappropriate calcium and silica metabolism.

Syphilitic teeth changes

There are many dental deformities in congenital syphilis (where the child inherits syphilis from intra-uterine infection during gestation). There is a defect of crown formation of teeth, especially between the period of birth to one year of age. Hutchinson's incisors are found in the majority, the teeth having eroded outlines that appear narrow and peg like. There are erosions of the occlusal areas of the other teeth with small bud like shapes. There is also a general hypoplasia of the teeth. In syphilis there is a gross incapacity of the higher spiritual blueprints to manifest into the physical tissues, as revealed by the deformed teeth.

Anthropological studies

These show that hypoplastic defects are very common amongst apes, monkeys and primitive stages of humanity (e.g. the Australopithecus and Paranthropus). The ego consciousness of apes is not individualised and would therefore find it difficult to maintain proper mineralisation of the teeth. The more modern and developed the human species the greater capacity the stronger ego incarnation has to provide a dense mineralisation.

Final thoughts

The final word rests rightly with Mercury and the mercurian planetary inhabitants. Although not visibly present, the mercurians are very much alive and present. The mythological god is typical of the race. Their powers of speed, agility and multi-dimensional travel are far beyond normal human comprehension. They are in preparing for the future evolutionary stages of Earth, when their planet will be asked to guide further flung energies from the cosmos into the Earth sphere and humanity. They will assist the supervision of a new race of humans, with psychic and spiritual powers built into the physical and genetic structure and from birth.

In one sense Mercury and its inhabitants function at the ultimate levels of service, guiding and integrating the myriad signals that require processing between Earth, humanity and the rest of the cosmos and spiritual realm. Without Mercury we would indeed be cut off, isolated and alienated as a race on a mass collective scale. This disease state is syphilitic and is revealed in the homoeopathic proving of the metallic remedy. As it is we live in an illusion of being separate from Source, but Mercury alongside many other beings has maintained the channels of communication during the dark ages of human history. As we pass into the re-birthing of Earth, Mercury presents opportunity and assistance to continue to develop our planet and ourselves.

Glossary

Adam Kadmon. The divine image and similitude of God within the human. It is the untainted blueprint within the human body makeup that is without karma, limitation, ageing, disease or degenerative processes. All human souls re-connect to this blueprint between their physical earthly lives in order to sustain the drive to perfection, the aim being to manifest the Adam Kadmon within the living physical form on Earth.

Adept. A person who has attained a certain level of spiritual initiation beyond simply mastery of the subtle and physical bodies. The soul has transcended the need to reincarnate into limited and karmic experience. The emotional body has transcended the need to have likes and dislikes. Consciousness has reached a universal level of functioning (the master level of enlightenment is at the relatively lower level of galactic consciousness). There are still initiations to complete until the next stage of Mahatmic and avatar consciousness, requiring further anchoring of cosmic consciousness and transcendence of emotional preferences into a state of no personal desire whatsoever.

Akashic records. A library of information within the fourth-dimension or astral plane, of all the experiences of each human soul across its past, present and future lives. It is not a fixed set of information but is constantly updated according to the changes made by a soul to its own memories and expectations.

Allopathy/allopathic. Any intervention or treatment within the sphere of modern westernised medicine – typically surgery and drug therapy. It is arguably unnecessary intervention and unnatural manipulation of the body.

Androgynous. The form where the nature of maleness and femaleness are within the same body. This was the primordial state before the formal segregation of the human race into male and female physical body types. There is thus perfect harmony within the being.

GLOSSARY

Angel. A particular class of spiritual beings that have not themselves undergone material incarnation into karma and limitation. Instead they assist the incarnated souls in countless ways – such as repairing and healing the physical-etheric bodies during nightly sleep of the soul; guiding Earth elemental forces and nature spirits in their interactions with humans; and supporting stuck fragments of a soul's consciousness in alternate and parallel realities within the multidimensional Earth.

– **fallen angel.** This coincided with a war in heaven between spiritual beings, and the fall of humanity. The state of being 'fallen' can only occur if there is a separation between the realm of spirit and that of matter. This separation is, however, ultimately an illusion. At multiple points during human evolution gods and other higher spiritual beings have been required to incarnate and copulate with early human forms and thus seed their genetic code into the human gene pool. Such beings have been referred to as fallen angels, gods of darkness, luciferic beings and so on. They have included various extra-terrestrial groups, including some from the star systems of the Pleiades, Sirius, Orion and Lyra.

– **guardian angel.** A higher spiritual being that assists the human soul in the management of the many alternate and parallel realities, which the soul experiences through the material plane. Each human soul has their unique guardian who usually transmits messages to the incarnated personality through the brow chakra. These messages help stabilise the personality when it feels negative emotional states (such as fear) during periods of crisis.

Aquarian age. The new age of consciousness for humanity, it is widely seen as a time for mass ascension on Earth. Many souls will succeed in overcoming the illusion of time and space, so as to consciously choose their journey on Earth. This will reduce the burden of karma, duality positioning and violence on the planet. Earth is progressively entering a finer state of vibration and astronomically is entering a photon belt where space is no longer seen as black, but as generally filled with light.

GLOSSARY

Archai. The beings inhabiting Mercury. They are adept at time-travel, especially into the past of humanity and our world, in order to retrieve experiences that require resolution. During their evolution there has been close interaction with the beings of Saturn.

Archangel. Angelic beings functioning close to the level of God. They supervise and harness epoch-making energies for whole worlds; i.e. they project qualities that imbue the development of civilisations for specified periods of time. Earth has recently left the epoch of time governed by Archangel Gabriel (who had imbued qualities of devotional and religious observance) and entered the epoch of Archangel Michael (who brings a need for freedom, liberty and the truth).

Arhat. Human beings who maintained a strong connection to the spiritual realm during the fall of humanity. This descent of human souls from the spiritual realm into the material was accompanied by a veiling of consciousness such that humans progressively fell out of harmony with the laws of spirit. The arhats maintained the ancient wisdom on behalf of future souls wishing to return into a self-realised and enlightened state. They were thus the ancestors of many of the spiritual masters and adepts of later ages.

Ascension. The descent of spirit into the material realm synonymous with the ascent of matter into the spiritual realm. Through this process the spiritual body (as a vehicle for self-consciousness or awareness) integrates more closely with the physical body. The physical and etheric bodies transcend the laws of earthly space and time, thus overcoming the ageing process and any degeneration. The disciple comes to anchor and manifest their immortality and divinity on Earth – and step out of karma and reincarnation. After completing ascension the disciple has a conscious choice as to where and when to journey after its allotted time on Earth, without the fetters of karma binding it into future obligations. The Earth is in a time of potential mass ascension, whereby many humans will achieve enlightenment. This will raise the vibration of the planet overall, assisting Earth itself to ascend into a pristine new and purified world.

A critical mass of 144,000 souls achieving self-realisation is required for this shift to become irreversible.

Astral body. The subtle body that, as part of the energetic makeup of the human being, governs the life of feelings, desires and sensations. It is the emotional body, but also having the much greater content of emotional experience arising out of all the incarnations of the soul. Thus feelings can transfer from the astral body into the lower conscious emotional body of the personality, giving it a sense of déjà vu or of having been there before. The nature of the astral body is to flow and even to fly. It connects to the physical body especially through the rhythm of breathing since its moves through the currents of airflow. It grounds into the physical body through the activity of the kidneys and adrenal glands. Thus heightened states of emotional fear can cramp the astral body and release surges of adrenaline from the adrenal glands, also leading to long-term kidney/adrenal damage. Most human diseases characterised by cramp, spasm and muscular tension (e.g. angina, irritable bowel syndrome, epilepsy etc.) are diseases of abnormal astral body flow within the physical–etheric bodies.

Asuri/Asuras' (pl.). These were rebellious gods and angels, cast out of heaven after an ancient war in that realm. These rebels have also been depicted as demons, fallen angels and the kabeira. They fell upon taking up pride and presumption, including a deep sympathy for the lot of ancient humanity (whom they viewed as cursed, but in doing so were obliged to share the karma of the fall from grace alongside humans). However the asuras were ancient gods of wisdom before their transformation into 'evil spirits' at perpetual war with the great god deities and faithful angels. 'Suras' is a Sanskrit term for gods, hence 'asuras', with the prefix 'a', indicates 'no-gods'.

Atlantis. The civilisation or race preceding our present Aryan one. The land mass is not strictly in the physical realm at present, but broadly equates to the region that is the Atlantic Ocean. It was submerged through karmic abuse of power, approximately 10,500 years ago. It was populated by the fourth root race of humanity, when the emotional body was developed within the human species (preceding Atlantis humanity had little sentient awareness of their feelings and emotions). It was also the development of the solar plexus chakra; hence problems often arise in this power centre from residual Atlantean karma. The key karmic imbalance during Atlantis was theft, including stealing other peoples' soul parts and trapping souls.

Bardo. The stage between earthly material incarnations during which the soul reviews its former life, within the astral plane of reality. During this experience images of the whole life are played back (often in reverse chronological order) and the soul perceives all the effects it had on others through the words, actions and thoughts of that life. This activates a sense of conscience and precipitates a desire to make amends, through the laws of karma, during the next incarnation. Many souls have phases of self-absorbed stagnation by becoming stuck in the lower astral plane in emotionally morbid problems still held in the memories of the former incarnation.

Bone-less race. The second root race within the present Earth chain of evolution. This ancient form of human had no mineralisation as such and therefore no skeleton. Their bodies were relatively watery and at best a firm jelly or a gel-like substance. The spiritual body had not yet descended sufficiently into the material realm to take hold of calcium phosphate or other mineral forces, thus being unable to incorporate these into the physical body. Beings were also relatively amorphous in their character, not yet able to assert themselves within any harsh terrain or situation. Souls were simply not firm or tough enough. The eventual development of mineralised and solid bone matrix to form an endoskeleton (internal skeleton) was required to strengthen human consciousness into individualisation and lower self egocentricity.

Cabalah. A language of light and vibration as used by spiritual beings to communicate with each other. This includes communication between humans in material incarnation with beings residing in the spiritual realm. All words are seen to have a numerical and energetic value (in the form of light, colour, tone, vibration or otherwise) and this can be calculated or deciphered through meditation. Many words have lost their ancient power over the last few hundred years through corruption by intellectual thinking and denial of the spiritual realm by the rational human mind. The cabalah seeks to remedy the lack of interaction between the spiritual and material realms through the language it depicts.

Chakra. A centre of energy flux that enables communication between the subtle bodies (spiritual, mental, astral and etheric bodies) and physical vehicle. They also provide portals for energy flow into and out of the being with respect to its environment. There are seven major chakras, called the crown, brow, throat, heart, solar plexus, sacral and base chakras. There are well defined pathways for energy flow between the chakras. Thus energy from the base and crown chakras inter-link, the sacral chakra connects with the throat, the solar plexus with the heart. The brow chakra serves an overall co-ordinating role. There are numerous minor chakras, such as at the back of the neck, hands, knees and feet etc. In the under-developed person, the chakras project energy out of the body from the front and the back (into the future and past time-lines respectively). The more developed spiritual disciple has spherical chakras that do not leak energy but retain it into a central column of energy. Eventually all seven major chakras unite into one chakra column, further clearing the illusion of separation since all levels of one's being then work in greater harmony.

alpha chakra. A junction point of energy between the physical and all the subtle bodies 15 to 20 cm above the head. It conducts the vastness and totality of one's spirit into the consciousness and energy field of the present incarnation.

alta major chakra. An energy centre situated at the nape or back of the neck. It often carries the energy of past life blocks to do with not manifesting one's thoughts into physical action. Many implants and etheric devices are situated here to block a person's ability to access their past lives. When it is opened through spiritual initiation, spirit guides can channel new insights in order to liberate the person from their past.

omega chakra. A junction point of energy between the physical and all the subtle bodies 15 to 20 cm below the base of the spine. It conducts the sum total of all past, present and future soul incarnations (within alternate and parallel realities) into the body of the present incarnation.

Channelling. The practice of opening one's energy field and consciousness to receive the energy, thought-forms and consciousness of higher spiritual beings (often known as spirit guides). In reality no human soul or personality unit is isolated. All beings are part of an infinite complex of all beings ever created, forming one cosmic unified consciousness. When this connection is felt again then the illusion of separation and the fall of the human soul into dense matter is overcome. A spiritual initiate has access to all knowledge across the whole time-line of creation and throughout the whole cosmos. This is part of the nature of God (omniscience or all-knowledge) and within all beings as their original spark of God-essence. Most humans do not realise that the thoughts running through their heads are directly perceptible to beings in the spiritual realm (thoughts often appear as structures and move faster than the speed of light). Also that most of the inspirational thoughts one has originate from spiritual beings liasing with one's higher self. Spirit guides often do not make themselves clearly perceptible; otherwise humans would enter states of glamour and dependence on their advice. They may initially depict themselves in role models, such as a Tibetan monk, a Red Indian native or western occultist or priest. Later the guide/s would lose this role and appear simply as beings of white light (which provides for greater flexibility). A common form of channelling in the past was trance mediumship, whereby the human channel (or medium) would partially vacate their own body to allow a spirit guide to take it over, thus transmitting messages verbally or through action to those sitting in séance around the medium. Upon return the medium could not remember the events or messages of the session. Conscious channelling has now superseded this, whereby the medium must learn to stay in their body and share their personal faculties with those of higher beings. This is now possible because humans have developed enough self-consciousness and Christ mastery to be able to communicate with spirit guides as equals.

Chi. This is the energy of the etheric body, and broadly equates with the concept of prana in Ayurvedic medicine or vital energy in homoeopathic philosophy. The etheric body has a complex structure, even more intricate than the physical body. Consequently there are many different forms of chi, such as food chi (chi derived from food digestion), gathering chi (a mix of inhaled chi and digested food chi), essence or jing chi (constitutional energy derived from one's parents and ancestors) or wei chi (a defence or immune system chi for protecting the body). Chi provides the energy for transport of vital fluids and all metabolic reactions. Problems in chi therefore lead to disease, such as stagnant chi flow causing chronic pain, or excessive and heated chi causing cramp and inflammation of organs etc. Chi can also be analysed according to its degree of yin and yang, which relates to polar qualities in the energy of receptive/passive and expressive/active dynamics respectively.

Consciousness. Another word for awareness, or sense of self. It is not a product of the physical body or even the higher subtle bodies. However it can only be perceived through its relationship with and expression through the bodies or vehicles of the self (i.e the spiritual, mental, astral/emotional, etheric and physical bodies).

– **Christ consciousness.** When a spiritual disciple activates Christ consciousness there is a deeper opening of the heart chakra, especially with golden flames igniting therein, and an activation of a special Christ Oversoul chakra above the crown chakra (and thus above the physical head). The present time on Earth of mass ascension of human souls is activating a collective Christ consciousness, whereby spiritual people around the globe sense a unity of energy and love (that in itself provides a wave of energy for mass transformation).

– **subconsciousness.** The level of consciousness that exists with reference to the subterranean realm of the second-dimension and the lower levels of the fourth-dimension. It often contains buried and past oriented experiences of souls. Each person does not, strictly speaking, have an individual subconsciousness; rather this realm can flow through each soul as a collective awareness. Humanity is fast becoming able to receive their subconsciousness and merge it into normal consciousness, although this process will complete only in future Earth rounds of evolution.

– **superconsciousness.** The level of consciousness that exists with reference to the higher spiritual realm, generally from the upper levels of the fourth-dimension to above. It is populated by spiritual guides, angels and extra-terrestrials, as well as housing the higher self or soul-spirit aspects of each human. Throughout this plane there is awareness of unity and the collective nature of spiritual intent, thought and emotional desire.

– **unconsciousness.** The level of consciousness that exists with reference to the first and lower levels of the second-dimensions. It is of the nature of metabolism and the many Earth processes that human souls cannot perceive directly, even though there are profound effects on humanity from these activities. This includes the activity of energy at atomic and subatomic levels of creation. In future chains of the Earth scheme there is the capacity to merge the unconscious with the normal conscious realm, at which point human souls will be able to alter the very forces of material creation.

Daimon (of fate). The individualised guardian angel that journeys alongside each human soul. This being assists the soul in maintaining the thread of consciousness between earthly incarnations, and supervises the movement of information between the various levels of consciousness (super-, normal-, sub- and unconsciousness). It also supports and maintains integrity of the physical and etheric bodies during the partial departure of the soul (along with its spiritual, mental and astral bodies) from these lower bodies during sleep. Eventually the human soul develops enough self-awareness and mastery to consciously control many of the above activities, but the daimon will still be needed for a long time by humanity in order to maintain the physical–etheric bodies and unconsciousness.

Devachen. The stage of rest for the human soul between earthly incarnations. It corresponds to the concept of 'nirvana' in Buddhist and Hindu philosophy, and is perceived as blissful and serene. This stage is particularly relevant for those souls that have developmental aspects within the lunar (Moon) chain of evolution, which preceded the present Earth chain. Devachen occurs after the lower bodies (physical, etheric and the denser parts of the astral body) have been disintegrated or re-processed in readiness for the next incarnation.

Dhyanis. Logoic (housing a collective identity) beings providing an energetic or astral double of themselves. This mirror image imparts the outer form or vehicle for individualised spirits to evolve through. The dhyanis had evolved during the previous three rounds of the Earth chain (during Old Saturn, Old Sun and Old Moon). Their astral double was transmitted to the first root race of humans in the present fourth round of the Earth chain of evolution. In essence they provide formative principles for Earth evolution and influence the various atoms that are in material existence, (which are not the same as the atoms understood by material science, but are energetic matrices for the different kingdoms of nature). From the radiation of the multi-dimensional bodies of the dhyanis came forth the elements making up the material realm (such as mineral, plant, animal, light, chemical ether radiation, etc.)

Dimensions (of reality). These are vibrational planes of reality, within which all beings reside and express their nature. They can be likened to the many levels of a high-rise building, with people living and working at each level. Each person will have a different vantage point and perspective upon looking outside the building; similarly consciousness is perceived in a different way when referenced from each dimension. All beings are effectively multi-dimensional, i.e. live throughout all the dimensions of reality. Dimensions are the means to structure or organise existence and allow one's divine nature to express itself. Using the dimensions, consciousness or spirit is able to function with the minimum of resistance. The Earth is now restructuring into a larger framework, which means it is changing from a predominantly third-dimensional existence into multi-dimensional reality.

– **first-dimension** is a passageway leading to a completion. The key energy in this dimension is completion. This shows that the Source or Creator has always been present and there is always something having existed. Therefore the beginning of a new life of creation involves the completion of something before. It is spatially related to be core of the earth.

– **second-dimension** is the beginning stimulation after something has been completed. There is a new emotional awareness and the key energy is of new beginnings. It is more active that the first-dimension. Spatially it relates to the realm of the subconsciousness and the elemental forces below the surface of the Earth.

– **third-dimension** houses matter as generally perceived and is the greatest densification of light energy. The key energy is magnification and this is the dimension Earth has recently left, where human souls felt secure and deeply stable. It imparts heaviness and has a slow vibration with space and time flowing gradually and in a linear way. Objects perceived in this dimension are almost frozen in space and time so as to become visible. Much creativity is possible because objects and experiences can be taken apart and studied in fine detail. This is how scientists attempt to understand the whole of creation by analysing the magnified manifestation of the third-dimensional reality alone. Spatially it relates to the surface of the Earth.

– **fourth-dimension** is called the astral plane and is essentially emotionally based. It is a realm of flow consciousness, often perceived when humans sleep (during dreams). Emotional energy radiates throughout this plane, causing attachment and repulsion between its inhabitants. This is a flow in all directions and in non-linear time and space, thus flowing faster or slower and in a more mobile way than the third-dimension. Resistance within the physical realm shows up more clearly as blocks to this flow. Souls must transit the fourth-dimension after death of their physical body, and much detritus or emotional junk lies in the lower levels of the astral plane from unresolved memories and experiences of past (and future as well as alternate) lives. Together the third and fourth-dimensions make up the lower creation realm where the game of separation can be conducted, where the illusion of good and evil can play out and individuals feel separate from spirit and from each other. As part of the ascension process all the lower dimensions will eventually become absorbed into the higher dimensions and cease to exist. The planet is currently vibrating at the middle and higher astral planes and is feeling more like a dream state for many humans. Dream themselves can change, such as more lucid dreaming and with a sense that there is not much difference between the dream state and the waking state.

– **fifth-dimension** brings awareness of being a master and a multi-dimensional being; becoming more spiritually orientated. The key energy is of structure. This dimension contains geometrical shapes such as large crystals with magnificent colours that interlock with each other. It holds the ideal blueprints and building blocks for creation of the lower dimensions. Many advanced human souls are now more consciously working within the fifth-dimension. It involves logical processes and higher concepts allowing for a greater creative potential to become manifest in the physical plane. The use of the fifth-dimension is important to anchor divine order, the divine plan and divine blueprints.

– **sixth-dimension** holds the templates for the DNA patterns of all types of species, including human kind. It is where light languages are stored, mostly of colour and tone and is where consciousness creates through thought. When operating sixth-dimensionally one is creating through consciousness without needing a vehicle for that consciousness. The key energy is of the ideal. It is the soul plane and contains the divine blueprints of collective consciousness for humanity. Everything happening to one soul is immediately known about and in agreement with all the other souls of this dimension.

GLOSSARY

The sixth-dimension is the electrical circuitry system that allows the divine currents to flow to the other dimensions. The sixth and fifth-dimensions make up the middle creation realm.

– **seventh-dimension** is that of pure creativity, pure light, pure tone and pure geometry. It is the last plane when one perceives oneself as an individual. There is a corridor between the sixth and seventh-dimension, which is a turnaround point, allowing for experiential objectivity. This is the realm where transpersonal positioning can truly begin to bring a greater spiritual outlook. The soul links to its monad or spirit through this dimension. There is a paradigm shift where one's perspective steps out of a sense of personality and looks at things in a more objective way.

– **eighth-dimension** is a plane for the group-mind or group-soul and is where one can touch base with the best part of oneself. It is characterised by the loss of sense of the I; however it is more likely that the human will fall asleep in this dimension because it is difficult to keep consciousness together within this group consciousness. Here all potentials are considered and explored. Much energy can be mixed to test the very many creative variables. The Source or Creator can therefore expand its understanding before setting up a plan of creation within the middle creation realm. It is a cosmic laboratory where other ideas from the co-creator level of the ninth-dimension are tested out; in other words each idea is stress tested in the eighth-dimensional laboratory.

– **ninth-dimension** is the plane of the collective consciousness of planets, star systems, galaxies and dimensions, it is difficult to remain conscious in this realm or to get a sense of self because one is so vast that everything is oneself. The key energy is co-creative. This is the co-creator level and has energies of ecstasy, pure joy and bliss. It interacts with all the other dimensions and is where divine energies communicate with the basic energy of the Creator. There is a feeling of transcendental consciousness through this dimension.

– **tenth- through twelfth-dimensions** make up the upper creation realm. The tenth is a source of the rays and home of beings known as the Elohim. New plans of creation are designed and then sent into the middle and lower creation realm. The eleventh-dimension is of pre-formed light, a point before creation and a state of exquisite expectancy. It is the realm of the being known as Metatron and of archangels and other akashics (primordial beings) for this Source system. There are planetary akashic records, galactic akashic records and akashic records for the entire Source system. Humanity is within one Source system of many Source systems, and each Source system is different. There are many universes within the many universes (in a many to many relationship, in other words everything interacts with everything). The twelfth-dimension is the one point where all consciousness knows itself to be utterly one with All That Is and there is no separation of any kind. After experiencing this realm one can never sustain the same degree of separation again.

DNA. The chromosomes are made up of DNA. It consists of two chains of DNA wound around each other to form a double helix, rather like a twisted ladder. The vertical support for each chain of DNA is a series of alternating sugar and phosphate groups, the sugar/phosphate backbone. The phosphate containing phosphorus is related to the Prometheus/Luciferic energy of the fallen luminaries (angels) who have provided a support system for human souls. Phosphorus carries light energy from the spiritual realm into the material. Sugar (as simple carbohydrate molecules) is a metabolic vehicle for ego/self consciousness to express itself in the physical body. Sugar is resonating with the mineral kingdom of the planet (note how crystalline sugar can appear in material form). Thus the sugar-phosphate backbone is literally a backbone or spine of ego forces upon which to hang the DNA molecules.

Ego. An individualised being with a personal sense of biography. It is another term for character, personality, self or 'I'. It is an organisation of personal perspectives and traits, and expresses itself particularly through the spiritual, mental and astral (higher emotional) bodies. All humans have an individual ego, which provides a sense of a personal journey to their consciousness. After the physical body is shed at death, the soul retains the characteristics of the ego developed during this previous incarnation and reviews its qualities so as to plan out its karma for the next incarnation. Progressively the lower ego during material incarnations aligns with the soul and spirit, until ascension is completed through a merger of these aspects of self.

Elementals. These are primordial beings that populate the etheric realm of Earth and are involved with the formation, regulation and maintenance of the etheric blueprints underlying all things manifesting into matter. They are also known as nature spirits or nature devas. There are many different elementals, specialising in the myriad types of energy, such as light ether, chemical ether, sound ether, warmth ether etc.

Etheric body. The subtle body that imbues the physical body with its sense of vitality. It is the seat of the metabolism and provides regenerative and growth capacities to the physical. It holds memories within a matrix of colour codes, geometrical shapes and sound tones. Etheric organs and tissues, the equivalent of those in the physical body, lie within it. Indeed loss or amputation of physical body parts can lead to symptoms felt within the etheric counterpart, such as phantom pains. The etheric body remains attached to the physical body until death of the latter, at which point it leaves with the soul and undergoes a partial degeneration. An etheric seed atom or residual part is carried by the soul into the next physical–etheric body at reincarnation, thus providing continuity of sub- and unconscious memory.

God. The supreme Creator or Source of the cosmos and multi-universes which were created out of his/her desire. There are three aspects to God's beingness, known as trinity.

– **Christ–God.** provides for the sense of mastery, perfection and an intimate relationship with the spiritual realm and its. See also 'Christ Consciousness'.

– **Father–God.** Carries the qualities of God's will, power and intent.

– **Mother–God.** Carries the qualities of God's love and nuturing intent.

Hades. The realm of the underworld, it is subterranean and houses soul fragments stuck in subconscious patterns between material incarnations of the soul. Mercury guides souls and their fragments to and from this realm.

Infinite soul. The state of soul when it merges with its cosmic monad or spirit. These are aspects of consciousness that transcend any limitation by matter, space or time and are not bound by the laws of karma and reincarnation. Such souls will incarnate on a planet during periods of great crisis and transformation, and impact it with world changing cosmic energy. They have included many of the avatars and spiritual founders of world religions. However Earth is reaching a level of ascension enabling infinite souls to incarnate that are more powerful than ever before.

Karma. All actions, words and thoughts expressed within the material realm create a resonant pattern of energy within the spiritual realm. Each soul thus weaves a destiny from such expression. The laws of karma affect everyone, and are not based on morality or punishment. They are the laws of compensation and adjustment of energy. Karma is inextricably interwoven with the laws of reincarnation, for karma creates a magnetic attraction and/or repulsion towards other beings and situations as a balance between the incarnations.

Kundalini. An energy which moves in a serpentine or curving manner and is the universal life-principle pervading all of creation. Without it there is no capacity for regeneration and re-birth. It is generally considered to reside coiled and hidden within the base chakra, but when activated it rises to activate the whole of the pranic tube and spinal cord. The spiritual initiate must learn to harness and thoroughly control this power in order to overcome the laws of reincarnation.

Law of similars. This is the basis to homoeopathy, and was developed as a systematic treatment by Samuel Hahnemann during the 1790s.

GLOSSARY

However it was accepted even before his days, for example Hippocrates (400 BCE), "By similar things a disease is produced and through the application of the like, it is cured". To treat with a medicine acting opposite to the direction of pathology does not invite curative participation of the patient's own vital energy, but can instead cause a suppression of the disease. In the words of Hahnemann: "Every medicine which, among the symptoms it can cause in a healthy body, reproduces those most present in a given disease, capable of curing that disease in the swiftest, most thorough, and enduring fashion".

Lemuria. The landmass that was home for the third root race of humanity. It was a huge continent stretching from the Indian Ocean to Australia and largely occupying what is now the Pacific Ocean, under which it is presently submerged. The highlands that have remained above water include New Zealand, the Fiji Islands and Papua New Guinea.

Logos/Logoi (pl.). A logos is a primary ray of energy used as a building block for the manifestation of spirit within matter. Generally logoi emanate as seven rays out of a prime logos. Each world, star, galaxy and universe has a logos or spiritual being ensouling it (within whom all other incarnated souls move and have their being). For example the logos of our galaxy is known as Melchior and of our Sun and solar system is Helios. The human celestial logos refers to the Adam Kadmon or primary human, a being that embodies all possible permutations and blueprints for the characterisation of human souls. All individual human souls evolve within the context of the Adam Kadmon as collective human consciousness.

Mahatma. A great being providing a vibrational scaffold for the entire cosmos. It forms the levels of vibration formulating the multiple dimensions of reality, the fabric underlying all universes, galaxies and solar systems, and the basis behind the infinite spectrum of consciousness from superconsciousness to unconsciousness. The Mahatma is in effect the architectural blueprint behind creation. It can also be used to refer to immensely enlightened beings known as avatars, whose conscious level of awareness stretches throughout the cosmos.

Manu. This is the divine thought-form running behind all events during one evolutionary round or cycle of time. It is the root-human or anthropomorphic personification of the human species during that cycle. Humans within material incarnation thus become a 'double' of their form within the spiritual plane. There are seven seed-Manus' within each globe or chain of planetary evolution, and thus seven rounds within each chain.

Medium See 'Channelling'.

Metatron. The archangel who is responsible for all light (manifest and unmanifest) within the cosmos. Everywhere there is light, there is Metatron. Since all material things are made from light energy, then metatronic energy pervades all of creation. Waveforms of this energy flow along the pranic tube (underlying the spinal cord) in a particularly sinusoidal manner. See also 'Pranic Tube'.

Miasm. An inherited or constitutional predisposition to certain modes of disease. It is generally considered to be genetic in basis and due to the pattern of diseases acquired from ancestors. For example a frequent incidence of tuberculosis within one's ancestors will create the tubercular miasm in the descendants; manifesting as weakness in the organs normally infected by tuberculosis (but without the microbial contamination) such as asthma and adrenal weakness. It is however also the history of disease along the time-line of incarnations of the soul, independent of the ancestors of any particular incarnation. Past life diseases can thus manifest as miasmatic tendencies in the present life.

Monad. An original spark of God. It can manifest as a whole solar system through to the tiniest atom. There are a definite number of monads created by God at the beginning (although it is also an unfathomable number). There is not a newly created soul for every baby that is born, rather each soul is part of a vast monad (which has become split into a number of souls). The personality of a human evolves to eventually merge with its soul, and then continues to evolve until it merges with its monad. This is the process of ascension.

Morphogenetic field. A modern term for the etheric field of energy around and through objects, all creatures, planets and stellar bodies. The Earth's field could reasonably also be likened to 'nature'. Within this field are stored memories, which can always be erased and re-written to suit evolutionary changes. Impulses from the higher spiritual realms interface with the physical or material realm through this etheric field.

Piscean age. Earth history is governed by macrocosmic events and the age of Pisces began about the birth of Jesus Christ (probably from 4 BCE when three planets were in conjunction in the constellation of Pisces) and has lasted two thousand years. The energy of this age imbued humanity with the forces of sacrifice, receptivity to religious and devotional energy, but also the desire to war with each other and rob their fellow human. Earth is presently in transition into the age of Aquarius, thus problems are surfacing in the conflict between the old obsolete Piscean energy and the new.

Pranic tube. The etheric counterpart of the physical spinal cord. It lies within a larger light-filled column running between the alpha and omega chakras. Coursing through the pranic tube are three waves of Metatron – the magnetic, electrical and gravitational. These provide for the material expression and manifestation of spiritual intent, desire and thought-form.

Ray. A basic spectrum of energy that pervades material manifestation. An understanding of the rays integrates the fields of astrology with soul psychology and human culture. All physical and subtle bodies, and each level of consciousness (from personality, through soul to monad/spirit) can be analysed by its ray make-up in an attempt to understand form and function. There are seven basic rays:

– **first ray.** Has the quality of will and power. It is particularly received by the crown chakra and is coloured red-white.

– **second ray.** Has the quality of love and wisdom. It is linked to the heart chakra and has an indigo colour.

– **third ray.** Has the quality of active intelligence. It is linked to the throat chakra and is coloured yellow.

– **fourth ray.** Has the quality of art and harmony through conflict. It is linked to the brow chakra and is coloured green.

– **fifth ray.** Has the quality of concrete knowledge and science. It is linked to the sacral chakra and is coloured orange.

– **sixth ray.** Has the quality of devotional love and idealism. It is linked to the solar plexus chakra and is coloured blue. It is the ray of the outgoing Piscean age.

– **seventh ray.** Has the quality of ceremonial order, magic and ritual. It is linked to the base chakra (but also the sacral) and is coloured violet. It is the ray of the incoming Aquarian age.

Root race. The predominant type and nature of the human race within each cycle or round of evolution within the planetary chain of rounds. There are seven root races represented by the seven rounds of evolution. Each root race develops a particular theme of evolution. A synopsis of each root race is as follows:

– **first root race.** Also known as the Polarean race, they were the ancestors of later lunar beings, they received energy directly from the Sun and had ethereal fiery bodies. They materialised by oozing out of the astral doubles of higher spiritual beings.

– **second root race.** Also known as the hyperborean race, they were produced by budding and sweating from the first-born race. Their spiritual and mental bodies were still very separated from their physical and etheric bodies (which were also not yet solidified fully). Some were gigantic in size.

– **third root race.** Also known as the Lemurian race. They segregated into the male and female genders of the human race and began egg bearing reproduction. Some were immense giants

GLOSSARY

and titans. They developed the faculty of speech and became more conscious the separation between the spiritual and material realms.

– **fourth root race.** Also known as the Atlantean race. They further developed gender characteristics and also their emotional nature. They generated heavy karma from abuse of technology and the theft of others' soul energies. During this race the Earth reached the densest point of its mineralisation and evolution.

– **fifth root race.** The present race of humans, it involved the development of the mind and increased capacity for learning. The middle point of this stage has now been passed.

– **sixth root race.** A future stage of humanity. This is on a parallel line of evolution with the second root race. There is great development of the forces of will and spiritual intent.

– **seventh root race.** A future stage of humanity. Beings will incarnate with full use of their spiritual powers within the material plane. There will be no further separation between the realms and the human race will be a race of adepts and spiritual masters.

Soul. The level of awareness or consciousness that lies between the immortal and transcendental nature of spirit/monad and the material nature of the incarnated personality. The soul mediates and communicates between the multiple personalities within incarnation, across space and time. It also mediates between these and the perfect state of spirit/monad, this latter being the state of being existing before, beyond and after all material incarnations and beyond all limitations in space and time. The soul is thus in a sense both perfect and imperfect. Many souls carry contracts and obligations within their soul records, defining their journey within patterns of karma and reincarnation.

– **soul fragment.** A part of the soul's consciousness that has become stuck within an unresolved experience. Invariably it is a part of the soul that is unable to let go of some emotional painful experience, or may have suffered some sort of abuse, or not have been able to forgive itself for some 'mishap' or abuse of its own powers. Often the person feels disconnected and alienated in some way. Ultimately all soul fragments must return to coalesce with the greater soul again, imparting a sense of emotional integration upon doing so.

Spirit. That element of consciousness that is before, beyond and existing after all limitation through matter has been overcome. It is that aspect of self that is perfect, immortal and aligned directly with God. The spirit or monad is directly infused with God's qualities of omniscience (all-knowing), omnipotence (all-powerful) and omnipresence (all-present). It is also the term for collective consciousness within the spiritual realm, and thus a harmonious unified state of shared awareness between all higher spiritual beings.

Sweat-born race. The second root race of humanity, when at one stage the beings reproduced by literally oozing new beings out of themselves.

bibliography

Albertus, Frater; 'Alchemists Handbook';
Samuel Weiser 1974

Bailey, Alice; 'Esoteric Healing Vol IV';
Lucis Press Ltd, London 1953

Baker, Douglas; 'The Jewel in the Lotus';
Douglas Baker "Little Elephant" 1985

Baker, Douglas; 'Esoteric Astrology';
Douglas Baker "Little Elephant" 1975

Beatty, Kelly et al; 'The New Solar System';
Sky Publishing Corporation 1999 and Cambridge University Press

Blavatsky, Helena Petrovna; 'The Secret Doctrine Vol I, II';
Theosophical Publishing House 1978

Clement, Stephanie Jean; 'Planets and Planet Centered Astrology';
American Federation of Astrologers Inc 1992

Csonka G.W. & Oates J.K.; 'Sexually Transmitted Diseases';
Bailliere Tindall 1990

Davidson, Alison; 'Metal Power';
Borderland Sciences Research Foundation 1991

Ellenhorn, Matthew and Donald Barceloux; 'Medical Toxicology';
Elsevier Science Publishing Company 1988

Harland, David M.; 'The Earth in Context';
Springer & Praxis Publishing 2001

Hillson, Simon; 'Dental Anthropology';
Cambridge University Press 1996

Husemann, Friedrich & Wolff, Otto; 'The Anthroposophical Approach to Medicine Vol I, II, III'; Anthroposophical Press 1989

Kerenyi, Karl; Hermes - 'Guide of Souls';
Spring Publications Inc 1976

Kranich, Ernst Michael; 'Planetary Influences upon Plants';
Biodynamic Literature 1984

Larousse, 'World Mythology';
Hamlyn Publishing Group Ltd 1965

BIBLIOGRAPHY

Mees, L.F.C.; 'Secrets of the Skeleton – Form in Metamorphosis';
Anthroposophical Press 1984

Merian, Ernest; 'Metals and their Compounds in the Environment';
VCH Publishers 1991

Morrison, Roger; 'Desktop Guide';
Hahnemann Clinic Publishing 1993

Pelikan, Wilhelm; 'The Secrets of Metals';
Anthroposophical Press 1973

Ridder-Patrick, Jane; 'A Handbook of Medical Astrology';
Arkana Penguin 1990

Scheps, Niek; 'The Trutine of Hermes';
Element Books 1990

Steiner, Rudolf; 'The Being of Man and his Future Evolution';
Rudolf Steiner Press 1981

Steiner, Rudolf; 'The Evolution of the Earth and Man and the Influences of the Stars';
Anthroposophical Press 1987

Steiner, Rudolf; 'From Comets to Cocaine';
Rudolf Steiner Press 2000

Treichler, Rudolf; 'Soulways- Developmental Crises & Illnesses of the Soul';
Hawthorn Press 1996

Twentyman, Ralph; 'The Science and Art of Healing';
Floris Books 1989

Vaughan, Valerie; 'Astro-Mythology';
One Reed Publications 1998

Vermeulen, Frans; 'Synoptic Materia Medica 2';
Merlijn Publishers 1996

Vermeulen, Frans; Prisma: 'The Arcana of Materia Medica Illuminated';
Emryss bv Publishers 2002

Vossius; 'De Origine ac Progressu Idololatriae' 1668

Waite, Arthur Edward; 'Hermetic & Alchemical Writings of Paracelsus the Great';
The Alchemical Press 1992

Wilkinson, Robert; 'A New Look at Mercury Retrograde';
Samuel Weiser Inc 1997

Worcester, John; 'Physiological Correspondences';
Swedenborg Scientific Association 1987

index

A

aborigines *221*
Achilles *80, 93*
Adam and Eve *131, 186, 190, 209*
 – Adam Kadmon *112, 208*
adenosine triphosphate *24*
adrenal gland *14, 163*
ageing *17, 56, 161*
Ahrimanic *147*
AIDs *142, 167*
akashic records *60, 119*
alchemy *4, 68, 105*
aluminium *24, 141*
amalgam *12, 24, 29, 141-5*
androgynous *106, 128, 165, 182-3, 187-8, 222*
Annubis *130*
antakharana *65, 202*
antibiotics *116, 168, 231*
Anubis *95*
apes *208, 216, 219, 239*
Aphrodite *106-7, 185, 194*
Apollo *81, 88, 97-101, 107*
Aquarian age *197*
Archai *41, 212-14*
Archangel Michael *79*
arhat *188*
Aries *75, 77*
Aristotle *122*
Asclepiads *108*
Asclepieion *108*
Asclepius *107-11, 159*
astral plane *26, 60-1, 119-20, 230*
Asuras *186*
Atlantis *112, 128-30, 143, 185, 196-97, 223*
Australopithecine *221, 239*

autism *140-1*
Autolycos *87*
axis tilt (planetary) *45*

B

bacterial fermentation *152*
bees *89*
birth control *195*
black magic *102*
blood groups *21*
bone marrow *177, 212*
bone-less race *185*
breathing *1-4, 10, 25-6, 126, 130, 169-75, 180-1*
brown fat *175*
budding *128, 187*

C

Cabalah *62*
caduceus *43-4, 83-4, 108, 161, 210*
calcium *127, 238*
Caloris basin *56*
cancer *30, 149, 161, 196-7*
carbohydrates *151-2*
carbon dioxide *169, 171-2, 175*
carbon monoxide *16*
Castor and Pollux *79-80*
cattle herders *101, 113*
celibacy *197, 202*
cell *21, 24-5, 148-51*
chakra
 – alpha *85, 210*
 – crown *128, 132, 204*
 – alta major *223*
 – brow *14, 127, 204*
 – throat *14, 124-7, 203-4*
 – heart *133, 203, 214*

INDEX

– solar plexus *129, 143-4, 203-4*
– sacral *107, 129, 142-3, 194, 203-4*
– base *163, 184, 204*
– omega *85, 210*
Christ *76, 84, 161*
– Christ consciousness *143*
chronic fatigue *10, 145*
cinnabar *20-1, 30*
clairvoyance *122, 127, 179*
clavicles *206-8*
clay *103, 147, 186*
consciousness
– subconscious *21, 25, 27-8, 52, 71, 76-8, 97, 113, 118, 128, 131-2, 200, 219-221*
– unconscious *2-3, 71, 86, 177, 214*
copper *23-4, 141*
crater *28, 45, 54-7*
crossroads *82*
cyanide *1, 15-17, 26*
cyclops *4, 222*

D

daimon *93-4*
Darwinian evolution *216, 222*
death *15-17, 60, 86-7, 92-8, 108, 119-21, 163, 174, 176, 179*
defence chi *149*
dementia *141-2, 167, 195*
depression *127, 155, 213, 229*
deva *84, 122*
devachan *119-20*
dhyanis *187*
digestion *138, 151, 153, 158*
dimension
– third dimension *60-1, 64, 87, 122-3*
– fourth dimension *26, 60-1*
– fifth dimension *26, 61, 120*
– sixth dimension *134*
Dionysus *106*
divination *88, 90*
duality *4, 75, 84, 150, 159, 163, 209*

E

Egypt *90, 94, 130-2*
– Egyptian Book of the Dead *94*
Elders *206-8*
elements *13*
elliptic orbits *45, 48*
Elohim *206-7*
EL-shift *208-9*
embryo *3, 115-6, 172-3, 178, 184, 188, 207-8, 233*
endoflagella *155-7*
Eros *104-5*

F

fall of humanity *4, 56, 131, 133, 154, 163-4, 208*
fanaticism *204*
Fates *88-9*
fats *151-2*
fertility *114, 175, 195*
fish *30, 106, 129, 165-6*
fission *186*
flagella *155-7*
forgetting *115-21, 220*
fungicides *30, 146*

G

Garden of Eden *190, 209*
Gematria *62-3*
Gemini *75-6, 79-80, 183*
genetic code *104, 112, 154, 159-61*
gestation *187, 233*
giants *188, 222-3*
gilgul *62, 67*
Gnosticism *73*
God self *63-4*
gold *1, 98, 132-8*
gonads *142, 203*
gonorrhoea *167, 195*
gravestones *113*

INDEX

Guardian Angel *88, 93*
Guardian at the Threshold *214*

H
Hades *94-8*
haemoglobin *16, 175*
Hall of Judgement *94*
hatmakers *82, 143*
heart organ and disease of *11, 167, 172-3 179-81*
Helios *34*
hell *21, 94, 96-7, 102*
Hermaion *102*
hermaphrodite *106, 112, 182-8, 194*
– Hermaphroditos *106*
hermeneia *105*
Herms *82*
Homer *80-1, 88*
Homo sapiens *222*
Hymn *80-1, 88, 101-5*

I
I Ching *159-60*
ibis *90, 94*
Illiad *80, 88, 93-4, 99*
immune system and diseases of *145, 149-51, 162-4*
implants *126*
infertility *175, 195*
inflammation *10, 149-50, 162*
information technology *61, 145*
iron *22-7, 57-9*

J
Jupiter *39, 80, 143, 177*

K
Kabeirean Mysteries *111-2*
kamaloka *119-21*
karma *66-7, 112, 129, 143, 165-6, 173, 209, 232*

Kepler's laws *48*
Keys of Solomon *206*
kleptomaniac *68*
Kumaras *64, 186*
kundalini *132, 184*

L
larynx *125-6, 129, 184-5*
lead *18-9*
lemniscate *211-2*
Lemuria *3-4, 57, 128-9, 165-6, 186-9, 196, 203*
Lethe *120*
liver *15, 31-2, 118-9, 143-4, 151-2*
Lord of Wisdom *92*
Lords of Form *176, 185*
lungs and disease of *2-3, 10, 16-7, 31-2, 126, 129-30, 168-75, 179-81*
lyre *102-4*

M
Mad Hatter disease *143*
magnetic field *57-9, 211*
Maia *79-81, 104*
marriage *178, 194, 198, 200-1*
Mars *24, 57-9, 77, 175-6, 223*
maya *121*
memory *27, 71, 104-5, 115-20, 134-5, 164, 174, 213, 220-1*
Mercurius corrosivus *11-12, 28*
Mercurius iodatus flavus *12, 15*
Mercurius iodatus ruber *15*
Mercurius oxycyanide *14*
Mercurius solubilis *4-6, 10*
Mercury fulminate *54*
mercury vapour lamps *24, 146*
merman *106*
metabolic system *172-3*
Metatron *85, 209-10*
methane *26*
miasms *154-5*

INDEX

microbes *10, 30, 150, 162-3*
mirrors *143-4*
Moon *26-7, 36-8, 52, 61, 76, 92-3, 134-5*
mucus *116, 149-153*
music *102-3*
mystery schools *130*
mythology *79,-82, 88-92*

N

natal chart *73*
necrosis *11, 31, 155*
Neptune *37, 39*
nerve-sensory system *135, 145*
nervous system *31, 82, 131-32, 146, 182-85*
 – brainstem *124-26, 183, 185, 223*
 – cerebrospinal fluid *107, 146, 164*
 – disease of *11, 142, 167*
Nile *90*
nominalism *122*
numerology *62-3*

O

Old Moon *27, 36*
Old Saturn *18, 36, 206, 212*
Old Sun *1, 26, 36, 40*
oomancy *90*
orbit *38-9, 42-52*
 – conjunction *45-6, 69, 72-3*
 – Mercury direct *73*
 – Mercury retrograde *69-74*
 – sidereal orbit *42, 52*
 – stationary points *69*
 – synodical cycle *46, 52*
oxygen *16-7, 25-7, 169-75*

P

parasite *153, 162-3*
parathyroid glands *124, 127*
parenthood *202*
parietal eye *4*

past life *126, 135, 142, 173-4, 212-3, 220-1*
perihelion *45, 47-51*
perspiration *10*
phallus *105*
pillar *63, 67*
pineal *3-4, 107, 128, 182-5, 199*
Pink disease *139*
Piscean age *197*
pituitary *107, 183, 199*
planetary ruler *74*
Pleiades *81*
poisoning *16, 29-33, 140, 143*
polygamy *195*
prana *17, 149, 169, 173, 176*
pranic tube *55, 85-6, 191, 203, 209-11*
preconception *202*
promiscuity *103, 129, 166, 190, 194-5*
proteins *149, 151-2*
protoplasmic cylinder *155-7*
psora *154-5*
psychopomp *96-9*

R

Rakshasas *186*
rays *112, 177, 197*
red blood cells *21, 175-8*
renal failure *31-2*
reproduction *184-9*
reptile *130*
rhythmic system *171-2*
root race *186-7*
rotation (planetary) *39, 47-54*

S

sal *135*
salamanders *17, 192*
salivation *10, 32, 139*
satellite *38-9*
Saturn *36-41, 127, 146, 177, 200, 212-4*
Scorpio *77, 186*

seed
– atom *119-20*
– Manu *186*
sexuality *10, 105, 128-9, 166, 189-90, 195-6, 203*
shapeshift *87*
Silenoi *106*
silver *27, 132-5*
skeleton and diseases of *11, 167, 206-14, 228-9*
sleep *60, 103, 108-11, 214*
snake *83-4, 108-10, 130-2, 209-10*
soul retrieval *196, 230*
spinal cord *55, 67, 85, 184, 208*
Spirits of Time *126*
Styx *120*
subsolar point *49*
sulphur *1, 20-1, 135-6*
Sun *1-3, 25-6, 38-40, 42-52, 82, 89, 92-5*
– Sun retrograde *48-9*
Sushumna *55*
sweat-born *185*
sycosis *154*
sympathetic nervous system *131-2, 185*
syphilis *139, 142, 155-68, 189-92, 239*

T

teeth
– adult teeth *216, 232-4*
– decay *10, 139*
– dentistry *141, 145*
– enamel *234-8*
– gingivitis *32*
– impacted *230-1*
– malocclusion *225*
– milk teeth *216-7, 228, 232-4*
– odontoglyphics *224*
– winging of teeth *227-8*
temperature *9, 22-3, 45, 52, 144*
temples of healing *107-11*
theft *99, 101-2, 144, 196*

thimerosal *140*
Thoth *90-94*
thyroid gland *14, 124-5, 127, 203-4*
tin *23-4*
titans *112, 222*
toads *192*
transcendental *124*
travellers *67, 102*
turtle *101-3*

U

ulceration *11, 31-2, 56*
ulcerative colitis *11*
umbilical cord *4, 27, 176*
underworld *21, 97-98, 130-1, 227, 229*
Universal Mother *93*

V

vaccination *140, 145*
vacuum *147*
Venus *39, 41, 59, 64, 76, 103-4, 200-1*
vertebral column *208-9*
Virgo *75-6*
volatility *20, 82*

W

windfall *101-2*

Y

yogic techniques *55, 172*

Z

Zeus *79-81, 100, 102, 104-5*

Forthcoming titles in the Homoeopathy of the Solar System series

The Sun and Gold

Venus and Copper

The Earth and Aluminium

The Moon and Silver

Mars and Iron

Jupiter and Tin

Saturn and Lead

Uranus

Neptune

Pluto

The Asteroids

Trans-Uranus

Vulcan

The Centaurs